This is a wonderful story that touched my soul. She spoke of her feelings and fears, giving them a voice. I believe that what she has shared on her journey can impact so many; for those who have touched her life and those she has touched, knowing that she truly understands and we are not alone."
- Jan Moffitt, MSW

I wasn't at all surprised when Debbie said she wanted to write a book to share her experience with others who are facing breast cancer. That is who she is. While others might feel isolated and feel that no one understands what they're going through, Debbie has consistently tried to put her suffering in a larger picture and learn from it in order to help others. I hope that others will find their inner fire burning within these pages of a woman's strength: who has been just flat out ferocious in her determination to survive."
- LouAnne Wise, MSW

"*Debbie's personal account of her emotional struggles is a wake-up call to us in the medical community. It puts a very brave face on this life-altering disease. She is a true survivor.*"
- Kathy Nomann, RN

SURVIVING BREAST CANCER

There Is A Child Within Us

Debbie Ziemann, RN

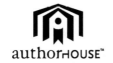

1663 LIBERTY DRIVE, SUITE 200
BLOOMINGTON, INDIANA 47403
(800) 839-8640
WWW.AUTHORHOUSE.COM

© 2005 Debbie Ziemann, RN. All Rights Reserved.

No part of this book may be reproduced, stored in a retrieval system, or transmitted by any means without the written permission of the author.

First published by AuthorHouse 07/06/05

ISBN: 1-4208-6630-3 (sc)

Library of Congress Control Number: 2005905939

Printed in the United States of America
Bloomington, Indiana

This book is printed on acid-free paper.

INTRODUCTION

Being diagnosed with breast cancer is a devastating experience. I want to share my story with all women; those who have survived, those who have been blessed with being free of not having to go through this experience, and those who have lost a sister, a mother, a wife, or a friend to breast cancer.

DEDICATION

I dedicate this book to all the women and their families who have survived breast cancer. I thank my husband, Wayne, for all the support and love that he gave to me throughout this experience that we have had to endure, and will endure for the rest of our lives. I also dedicate this book to my sons; Brady, Evan , and Aaron, for always being there for us;

To Diana Bool, LouAnne Wise, and Jan Moffit; who as dear friends shared this journey with me.

To Dr. Geoffrey Leber; who, through his compassion, kindness, patience, and understanding, was always there to listen and validate my feelings. Dr. Leber helped me through one of the most difficult times of my life.

And, I also want to thank all my "special friends" at Hospice of Arizona for listening and giving me the support I needed, as I struggled through this experience.

FOREWORD

When you have been diagnosed with breast cancer, the journey just begins. There are many fears which you must face; much pain and sadness. Even though it is a body part that we lose, there is a lot of grief involved. Every one will go through the grieving process differently. How we fight to get through the grieving process will be different for each person.

Life is unfair! There is never a right time for something to happen. But, there is always a reason for the things which happen in our lives. We may not be able to understand at that moment, but time will show us the reason. We have to learn to enjoy each moment, taking one day at a time. We have to allow ourselves to have bad days and to cry. It is part of the grieving process.

"Bad Things Do Happen To Good People," and we need to use any unfortunate event in our lives to teach us that each day is a Gift. Only then can we truly see the beauty of each moment, each experience, and see the extraordinary in the ordinary.

We often take for granted the most valuable gifts that we have: spouse, family, and friends. We are so consumed in this busy world with making a living that we forget to make a life. We need to learn to enjoy the little pleasures of life: a walk in the park, watching the sunrise and sunset, holding hands with our spouse, and enjoying the beauty around us. This journey that we take with a life-threatening disease is the start of a new life. Our priorities change, and we no longer take for granted those things that are most precious to us. We learn that life is a gift and we learn to live it joyfully!

TABLE OF CONTENTS

Introduction	v
Dedication	vii
Foreword	ix
1. The Beginning	1
2. The Consultations	11
3. Multiple Surgeries and Complications	31
4. Anxiety of Chemotherapy	65
5. After the Treatment, the Struggle Begins	85
6. State of Mind	93
7. Life Will Never Be The Same	107
8. Struggling Through the Grief	117
9. A Special Christmas, 2004	127
10. Rediscovering Myself	133
11. I'm Okay!	145

Chapter One
THE BEGINNING

*M*any do not believe in "love at first sight". I was one of them, until I met my present husband. I was a single mom, for 21 twenty-one years, raising three sons. I moved to Arizona in 1997, bought a home, and began working as a Director of Nursing in a Long Term Care/Rehabilitation Center. Then I made a career change in 2001.

I went to work for Hospice of Arizona. I assisted patients and families through the end-of-life process. The philosophy of any hospice program is to provide comfort and dignity. Hospice is a very rewarding healthcare career. It is not for everyone, however. We have a gift to offer our patients and families: accepting them for who they are, not passing judgment, and assisting with education, emotional, and spiritual support, and physical comfort.

But, our patients and families also give us a gift; they share their lives and their journey with us.

I was one of those people who searched for companionship on the Internet, being very careful where and when I met men. In May of 2000, I came across a bio, and my heart started to race. I said to myself, "Oh, my God, this is the one." I wrote an email, and within two hours he wrote back. He was out of the country and would be back in two weeks, and wanted to meet with me. We wrote to each other every day while he was gone. I remember hurrying home from work, anxious to see if he had written, and would write back immediately. On June 12th, we were to meet at Old Chicago. I sat and waited; he was late. I was ready to leave, when this tall man came in and said, "Are you Debbie?"

I got up and said, "Yes." We shook hands and I felt my knees weaken. There was tenderness in his hands, a beautiful smile, and sincerity in his eyes. My heart was racing; I was so nervous. I could not help but hope and pray that he was feeling the same way. We had a wonderful lunch and he asked to see me again!

Our relationship grew, and we both knew that this was "love at first sight"! We had some difficulties, as any couple does in the beginning of their relationship. But, we found out that we did not want to lose one another. We were each who the other had been searching for, all of our lives: someone to grow old with and share the little pleasures of life with. The summer of 2002, we decided to get married that December.

We went to an antique shop, and we saw a 1930's satin lace wedding gown there. It was just beautiful! It was just perfect! But, I was sure that it would not fit, so we left without it. I told my best friend, Jan, a social worker from the hospice that I had worked with for two years, about the dress. We decided to go together to the antique store and see if the dress was still there. I could not believe it! It was right where I had seen it. I tried it on, and it fit! Jan and I both started to cry because we both knew that this was meant to be. I was meant to wear this dress on our wedding day.

You can remember all the preparations that go into a wedding: the food, music, accessories, and flowers. We were getting married in our back yard, on December 23rd. In Arizona, the weather should have been in the 70s, but instead it was in the 60s, and cold and raining. RAIN! An Italian good luck sign of wonderful times to come!

We got married in our living room beside the Christmas tree. My youngest and oldest sons gave me away. Evan, my second son, provided the music. Evan and Brady are chefs, so they cooked all the food, and it was delicious. We had a wonderful time. We were married and got to celebrate Christmas with my sons, all at the same time. Such a beautiful gift!

We went through a lot of emotional stress the following year: Wayne traveled, installing and repairing newspaper presses, and he was only home every other weekend. In October of 2003, we went on vacation and found out that his identity had been stolen when we went to use his credit cards. He, then, became a victim of age discrimination with the company that he was working for. In February of 2004, he developed pneumonia, and was home for several weeks.

Because of the illness, the stress of being away from home so much, and the problems with his employer, his diabetes became out of control. The doctor advised him that he should no longer travel. After much discussion, he resigned in March of 2003. He was anxious to find another job. In March, he was called for an interview as a electrical maintaince supervisor. It went very well, and he was hired.

I truly believe that everything happens for a reason. Although, at the moment when something bad happens, we do not understand why. For a long time, Wayne could not understand why everything seemed to be going wrong in his professional life. But we soon found out why:

We were about to be told that I had breast cancer.

March 1, 2004

I had my annual physical, which included a mammogram. Two weeks went by, and there was a message on our answering machine that the doctor wanted to see me to discuss the results. My heart just sank down to my toes. I knew then that this was not going to be good news. Being a positive person, I told my husband that it was probably just because there were fibroids, and that she wanted to do more testing.

They got me in right away, and I was to have an ultrasound and a needle biopsy. I called and scheduled those procedures. I went to have those procedures done and had a very bad experience at the breast ultrasound company. They had no compassion or understanding of the anxiety or fear of the unknown. They argued with me about why I was there. They would not tell me what they found. The radiologist who spoke to me said that I needed to have a biopsy, and if time was of the essence, they may be able to schedule the biopsy the following week. I told her that I was hoping to have it done that day, like it was scheduled.

She said, "So would every woman sitting in the lobby."

I was angry! I wrote a letter to them and sent a copy to my nurse practitioner about their unprofessional behavior and attitude. There was not one sign of understanding of the emotional factors involved, or the anxiety that my husband and I were going through. I called my FNP, and got a list of surgeons to see, so that I could consult with them, instead of waiting to have a needle biopsy. Out of eight surgeons that were recommended, there was an unknown force which lead me to I decided on Dr. Robert Leber. Little did I know at that time, but his son, Dr. Geoffrey Leber, a plastic surgeon, would become part of my support system.

It is very important that you are comfortable with your surgeon. He must treat you as a person, not a surgery or disease. He, or she, must take his, or her, time with you, and allow you to talk about your feelings, worries, concerns, and fears. He must show kindness, compassion, and allow you to cry. He needs to be able to share your journey with you.

God's Boxes

I have in my hands two boxes
Which God gave me to hold.
He said, "Put all your sorrows in the black box,
And all your joys in the Gold.

I heeded His words, and in the two boxes
Both my joys and sorrows I stored.
But though the gold became heavier each day
The black was as light as before.

With curiosity, I opened the black
I wanted to find out why.
And I saw, in the base of the box, a hole,
Which my sorrows had fallen out by.

I showed the hole to God, and mused,
"I wonder where my sorrows could be?"
He smiled a gentle smile and said,
"My child, they are all here with me."

I asked God, why He gave me the boxes.
Why the gold and the black with the hole?
"My child, the gold is for you to count your Blessings,
The black is for you to let go.

- Author unknown

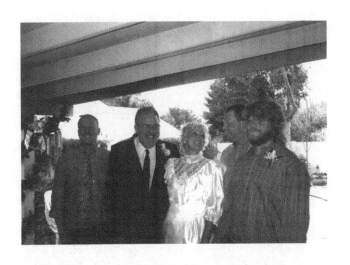

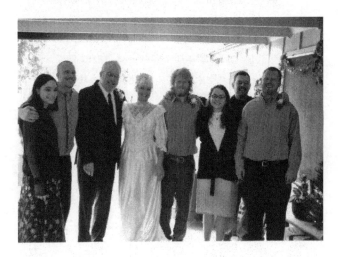

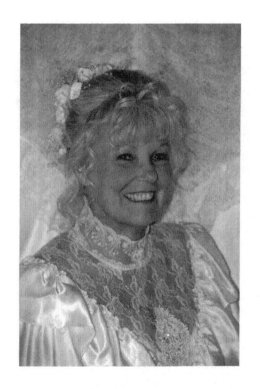

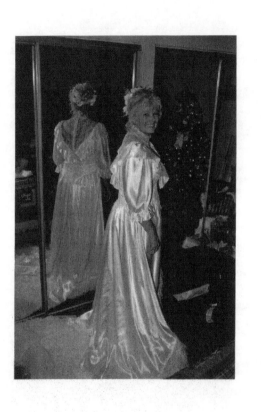

Chapter Two
THE CONSULTATIONS

*T*owards the end of March, we went to see Dr. Robert Leber. I took the ultrasound films with me because he wanted to read them. We sat in the waiting room, anxious and very nervous. We were called in and we went into an exam room. The medical assistant took a brief history and then I had to disrobe and sit on the exam table. We saw all of his certificates hanging on the wall from all the medical schools that he had attended, and his board exams. We were impressed, and our comfort level with the choice of surgeon rose to alleviate some anxiety that we may have had with the choice of surgeon. Dr. Robert came in and introduced himself to both of us. He is an attractive man, kind, and compassionate.

He took a medical history and then did an examination of my breast. He spoke very softly, and looked at the both

11

of us, and told us that the breast needed to be removed. He explained that because of the location (which was under the breast and involved the nipple), a lumpectomy was not an option because he would have to remove two-thirds of the breast. He excused himself and left us alone. I got off the table and went to my husband and began to cry. He held me tightly and told me that it would be all right. I could feel his fear.

Thoughts just raced through my head. I was afraid! My mother had died of cancer when she was fifty-four. I was afraid that Wayne would fall to pieces. He is my protector and I knew that he would feel inadequate because he would not be able to fix it. I didn't want to lose my breast; no matter what people think, it is a part of who we are. I even thought that maybe Wayne would leave me because I would no longer be physically attractive to him. I knew in my heart that would never happen, but it is still a normal fear that everyone goes through.

Dr. Robert came back in and we were still holding one another. He said, "I caught you." I smiled and told him that we had only been married fourteen months. There was silence from him. He again examined the breast and had me stand. He explained that I definitely needed to have a mastectomy. He said that he would do a centennial biopsy as well and remove the lymph node.

From the results, he would know whether he would have to remove any more nodes. He strongly felt that I was a candidate for a TRAM-flap reconstruction. He gave us all the options, however; a TRAM Flap which would allow me to have chemotherapy, or I could have implants, which would have to be done after the chemotherapy. He said that I would have to take Tamoxifen, but if I did need chemotherapy, that would increase the survival rate to 92%.

He told us that his son, Dr. Geoffrey, was a plastic surgeon, and they had been practicing together for some time. He smiled and said that in the beginning, he didn't think that it would work, but that it had turned out very well. He had me get dressed. Then, we went out, and he met us at the desk. He said that he would give my medical file to his son and that I would need to make an appointment with him. Then Bonnie would coordinate the surgery because of their different schedules. Luckily, we were given an appointment for the next week to see Dr. Geoffrey. I was impressed with the concern and the urgency that they showed to have the appointment made quickly. It gave me some relief to know that there was a sense of urgency because some physicians take their time, and then it can be too late.

As we walked hand in hand from the office, I began to cry. Wayne's hand was shaking. I felt that my world had been turned upside down. We had just been married a year. I had been single for twenty-one years and finally found someone whom I felt I had waited a lifetime for. I had started a new life and it was being snatched from me! He comforted me and said that it would be all right, and that he would be with me through this, and we would have a long life together. We drove home in silence. Later. sitting on the couch, I told Wayne that he would need to be strong for me and I would be strong for him.

Being a registered nurse has its advantages, but it also has its disadvantages. I knew that the success rate for breast cancer has increased dramatically over the years. However, working in hospice, we only see the unsuccessful outcomes, and images of patients I had taken care of through the end-of-life process went through my mind.

My mother, who, at the age of thirty-two, was diagnosed with terminal ovarian cancer, went through my mind. She had multiple surgeries, several courses of chemotherapy, and complications from the chemotherapy.

SURVIVING BREAST CANCER

She finally passed away when she was fifty-four, in October of 1984. I recalled her misery, but I also remembered her strength and determination to live. I was not sure that I could endure what she had.

That evening, Dr. Geoffrey called and introduced himself. He said that his father had given him my records, and that he was reviewing the medications I was taking. He asked if I was still taking the Cenestin (hormone replacement). I told him that I was, and he instructed me to stop. He said that he would see me next week, and told me not to worry, and that everything would be all right. Once again, I felt relieved, knowing that I had made a good choice in surgeons. His caring attitude and compassion were both apparent as he spoke to me. It would be later, that I would tell him that I was drawn to him and his father and did not understand why at the time. It was weeks later, that I realized that God was directing me, because I would need his compassion and strength.

We went to see Dr. Geoffrey the following week, and once again, we sat in the waiting room, anxiously holding hands. I filled out another medical history and insurance forms, as we all have done many times before. We were taken into an exam room, and I was given a full gown to put on, and I sat on the exam table.

Dr. Geoffrey knocked, came into the room, and introduced himself to both Wayne and me. He sat down and talked to us about what his father had told us. He then proceeded to do an exam of the breast; he had me stand in front of him so that he could look at my abdomen. How embarrassing that is! Standing naked in front of a strange man, baring your personal parts, sharing something that only the person that you are intimate with has seen and touched. I have always been self-conscious of my body, and to have a stranger, even though he is a surgeon, see me without clothing was humiliating. He told us that a TRAM flap would be effective and explained the procedure. He also gave us all the options, as his father had done. I looked at Wayne and told him that I would rather have the TRAM flap rather than to go through more surgery later. Wayne said that I should do whatever I thought would be best. He had no medical knowledge about these things and so he was leaving it all up to me.

I had to go into another room with Dr. Geoffrey, where there was a drape. He asked me to remove the gown, and he gave me a G-string to put on. He said that he would be back. Reluctantly I did what I was asked .

SURVIVING BREAST CANCER

I put the gown on and waited for him to return. I never expected what was to come next. He returned with a camera! He sat on a stool and told me that he was going to take pictures and do some drawings. I stood in front of him, baring my imperfect body, looking up at the ceiling, with tears running down my cheeks. Holding my arms in the air, he took pictures, measurements, and manipulated the fat on my abdomen. He asked if I was all right; I told him that I was just embarrassed.

Then, I had to stand in front of the blue drape. Facing him he took pictures, standing to the left, with my arms up, and then bending over. Then, he asked me to turn around, to the other side, and he repeated the process of taking the pictures again. I was so self-conscious about how I look without clothing. I never allowed anyone to see me naked before. I have always been heavy and after having three babies and losing one hundred pounds, I had a lot of excess fat and skin. Wayne was the only one that ever saw me naked. He never made me feel self-conscious about how I looked.

I had never allowed my first husband to see me naked. I dressed behind closed doors and took my shower with the bathroom door closed. I am sure that must be a shock for some, but, I believe that it came from the way I was raised as a child. And as I grew older, I was able to accept how I looked physically and was no longer embarrassed.

17

Debbie Ziemann, RN

He then helped me put the gown back on and had me sit on the table. He explained that he wanted to first revascularize the abdominal wall to ensure that there was adequate blood flow when he did the TRAM-flap. He then told me how that would be done; he would remove a large section of the abdomen and pull it up under the chest wall to make a flap, reconstructing the breast. The breast would be large and that would be revised later so that both breasts were symmetrical. He explained all the possible complications. I already knew all the complications, as a nurse, but it frightened me even more. The fear of the cancer having spread to the lymph nodes was one of my biggest concerns. I told him that I understood, but that it didn't alleviate my fears. He promised me that he would take good care of me and that he would see me through this.

The first surgery was scheduled for the 21st of April, at the outpatient surgicenter next to his office. When we were ready to leave, Bonnie said that we had a really good surgeon and that he would take good care of me. She said that everything would go well and that I would be all right. It was apparent to me that the office staff enjoyed working for these two physicians and that they had a lot of confidence in their abilities. Although that was a comfort, we were still very anxious.

Walking out of the office, I was crying. I was so embarrassed from standing in front of a stranger, totally exposed, and having pictures being taken in different positions, showing all the stretch marks and sagging skin. I was afraid that he would be thinking how disgusting it was and wondering why I hadn't taken better care of myself. It wasn't until later that I realized that Dr. Geoffrey is an artist. He takes pictures, drawing on your body, and then surgically creates a masterpiece: a Michelangelo of the twenty-first century!

The following week, I had all the pre-operative lab work, including a chest x-ray and electrocardiogram, and then went to his office after work. I was taken into his office, where he explained all the consent forms, and the complications. He asked if I was sure that this was what I wanted to do, and I told him that I felt that this was the best option for me. Later, I thought that he was trying to talk me out of this procedure because he was not sure that it would be effective. Later, I would learn from him that he would not have agreed to the TRAM-flap if he had not thought that it would work.

I realized that there was something important that I needed to complete. There is something that we all put off until we have to: setting up a living will and a durable

19

power of attorney. We put these off, because it makes us think about our mortality, but I realized that no matter how difficult it might be to complete these, I needed to do it. I asked LouAnne, a social worker, to help me with this. She brought the forms to work and we completed the living will. I knew that I needed to make sure that my husband knew that I did not want my life prolonged for any reason. We had talked about this before, but he didn't understand why I did not want any extraordinary means to support my life.

Completing the power of attorney was more difficult. I asked LouAnne if she would do that for me. She agreed most graciously after making sure that I did not want one of my sons to be designated. I told her that I did not want my husband or my sons to be in a position to make the decision of stopping treatment or life support, in the event that I could not make that decision. I wanted someone who could give them the support they needed and respect my wishes. I didn't want any of them to have any guilt for allowing me to pass from this life to another.

I had another difficult mission to accomplish. I have a sister that I have not communicated with for several years. I had learned that she was angry with me but was not sure why. I decided to write to her and let her know what had happened. I needed to mend the gap that had come between us. Even though I knew there was a possibility that I would not be able to restore our relationship, I had to try. I would have to have closure, so that I could have peace, knowing that I had done what I could to resolve the hurt that we caused one another. We now write one another, but there is still some mending to complete.

I had not spoken to my father for several years, either. He had divorced my mother in her greatest time of need, when she was going through chemotherapy, and he divorced his daughters, also. I wrote to him, to let him and his wife, Bonnie, know that I was having a mastectomy for breast cancer. Surprisingly to me, they wrote back and now we are keeping in touch.

I was also concerned about the financial hardship that we would have. We talked about closing Wayne's 401K, which would help us while I was off for twelve weeks. We decided to cash it in and pay the penalty. Adding to all the stress and anxiety that we had about the diagnosis and upcoming surgeries, the check never came. The bank said that it was mailed and returned signed. We filed a fraud claim, and the bank then wired the money to our account, the day of the mastectomy.

We realized that if Wayne had remained on his past job, traveling, I would have had to go through this alone. He would not have been able to take the amount of time off from work that we would have needed. I told my husband that he had to go through all that he had with his previous job so that he would be able to be home with me, and we would be able to go through this together.

I could not have gone through this alone, without him.

Now the hard part came: I had to tell my sons. I had put it off long enough, and time was moving quickly. I called the youngest, Aaron, first. He would be twenty-six in May and was living in Ohio. I told him what had occurred. They had found a mass and I needed to have surgery. I told him about seeing the surgeons and what the plans were and when I would have surgery. I told him that they were 90% sure that I would not have to have chemotherapy.

He was quiet, and then he asked how I felt about this. I told him I was all right and that it was caught early so the prognosis was very good. I tried to remain as positive as I could and not let him hear the anxiety that I felt deep within me. He asked how Wayne was doing

SURVIVING BREAST CANCER

with this news, and I told him that he was scared but we were being strong for each other. Aaron's voice started to shake and I could hear him starting to cry. I reassured him that it was going to be all right, and he needed to keep a positive attitude and say a lot of prayers. He wanted to know if I wanted him to come out and I told him not yet. Maybe, when I had the second surgery. But, we would call him and let him know how I was doing. I told him that I needed to call his brothers, so we said good-bye and love you.

I called Evan, the second son, who lives in northern California. He always calls me "Mommie". We talked a bit about what he was doing, his work and new girlfriend, Carli. Then, I broke the news. He was full of questions. I answered them to the best of my ability, and told him everything that I had told Aaron. He also wanted to know how Wayne was handling this, and once again, I told him that he was scared but was being strong and supportive. He asked if I wanted him to come, and I told him no, that I would let him know how things went, and if we needed him to come, I would let him know. We would call him often to keep him informed.

Although it was difficult telling the two youngest sons, the real difficult call was now coming, to my

23

oldest, Brady, who will be twenty-nine in May. He lives in Sacramento, with Lindsey, his girlfriend. He had some really difficult times over the past several years, and we had become really close. I knew that he was not going to take this news very well at all. And I was right! He had just gotten home from work, at a catering business, and talked about what had been happening in his life. I then told him that I had something that I needed to tell him. He knew right away that something was wrong.

He was angry! Not at me but at the fact that this was happening. He raised his voice so I started talking softly so that he would calm down and listen. I explained everything to him. I could hear him start to cry. And then suddenly, he didn't want to talk any more. I told him that it was going to be all right, and that he could come if he wanted to. I thought that would make him feel more at ease, so that he could see that it was going to be fine. He said all right, and we said our good-byes and I love yous.

I sat down beside Wayne and leaned against him. As he held me, I began to cry. I told him that I was not angry. That I was not asking "Why me" because why *not* me? But, I was asking "Why now?" Why now, when we are newlyweds? Why now, when our life together is just starting? There were no answers. And once again I said, "Everything happens for a reason, we just don't know what the reason is for this to have happened. There are many possible answers; some could be right or wrong. Maybe all of them are right, or wrong, but right now, it does not matter. What matters is that it has happened, and that there is a reason. Whether we ever realize what that reason is, is a matter to be seen.

The next step was to tell my team at Hospice of Arizona. I told them that I had been diagnosed with breast cancer and would be having surgery on the 16th of April. There was silence. I explained some of my feelings and that Wayne and I had been making silly remarks about the reconstructed breast. It was our way of dealing with our fear and the uncertainty of what might come. I found myself crying, but acknowledging that I would be all right, and the positive attitude that the physicians had about the results. I told them who would be taking over the team, and I would keep in touch with them, and with that, I closed the meeting. They all came to my office afterwards and hugged me; letting me know that if I needed anything at all, to call them. They would keep us in their thoughts and prayers. I was smiling through the tears.

On that Friday, my co-workers took me to lunch. We were laughing and having a wonderful time. They then gave me a gift bag and a card. There was a nightgown, puzzles, word games, and a couple of Teddy Bears, and an angel. The thoughts that they wrote to me in the card gave me strength and courage. Through tears and laughter I knew once again that everything would work out. I am a strong person, a determined individual with the patience of "Job", but I would soon find out that I was not as strong as I had thought, and that I was going to have my patience tested.

At times, I cried when we were lying in bed. I was worried about looking mutilated, worried that Wayne would think I was less than perfect, or that he would find me repulsive and would not want to be intimate any longer. I was afraid that he would find me physically so repulsive that he would leave and want a divorce. Those are normal thoughts, and have been actual events in other people's lives, and I did not want to go through that. If it happened, I didn't know if I would be able to go through the rest alone.

I am sure that when I told my husband about those thoughts, he was probably hurt, although he didn't say so. He reassured me that he was "with me for the long haul", and that he married me for who I am inside. He reassured me that it didn't matter to him if I had one, or two, breasts; I was the same person he had married. I didn't know then that it would be me who was afraid to be touched, or to be seen without clothing, and with no hair.

I don't believe in Miracles.
I rely on them!
Life may not be the party we hoped for,
But while we are here,
We might as well dance.
Life is not a journey to the grave
With the intention of arriving safely,
In a pretty and well preserved body,
But rather to skid in broadside,
Thoroughly used up, totally worn out,
And proclaiming loudly –
"WOW – What a Ride!

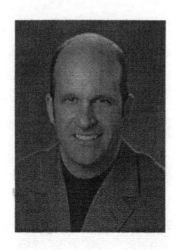

Above: Dr. Geoffrey Leber

Below: Dr. Leber and Staff

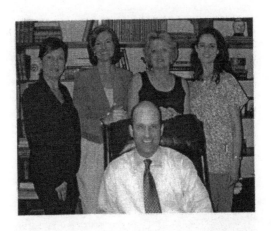

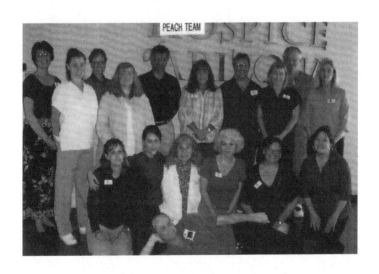

Chapter Three
MULTIPLE SURGERIES AND COMPLICATIONS

*I*t was April 21st, the day of the first surgery in preparation for the mastectomy. I had Wayne drop me off at the surgicenter and go to work. I didn't want him to take the day off because it was a new job; he had just started. I didn't want him to put that in jeopardy. Jan met me there, and we waited in the lobby for them to take me into the holding area. This surgery was not the one that I was concerned about. It was scheduled for two hours, and then after an hour in the recovery room, I could go home.

The nurse came, got us, and took us back. She completed a small history, made sure that I had had nothing by mouth after midnight, and then gave me a gown and slippers to change into. I then went to the gurney where Jan was waiting. The nurse, Patty, came and said that she was going to start an IV and then put on some anti-embolism stockings with alternating pressure hose. The anesthetist and Dr. Geoffrey would come see me before the surgery.

When the nurse was through with me, Jan and I talked. She gave me a worry stone to rub. I noticed that I was furiously rubbing the stone. I was more nervous than I had thought. She told me to take deep breaths and think of the color green. Closing my eyes, I thought of a green golf course. Taking a deep breath, I saw the mist flow into my body and upon exhaling, small balls of light left my fingers and toes. She had me concentrate on the color purple and white, surrounding me, giving me a feeling of peace. It worked! I was relaxing, and there was a sense of peace within me.

Dr. Podenko came. He asked if I was nervous and I had to say yes; it was that apparent. He said that he was going to give me some medication to relax me, and that when he took me into the surgical suite that he would put me to sleep and I would not remember a thing. I laughed and told him to "bring on the drugs!" He smiled and laughed. Then Dr. Geoffrey came. I introduced him to Jan and told him that he could talk to her when the surgery was over. He saw that I was anxious. He took my hand and said that everything would go well, that I would be in recovery for an hour or two, and then I would go home. I hugged Jan, and she told me that I would be just fine. And she went to the waiting room.

Dr. Geoffrey, Dr. Podenko, and the circulating nurse took me into the surgical suite. I moved over to the surgical table, not remembering how cold those rooms could be. The nurse brought a warm blanket. Dr. Geoffrey came and stood by my side and held my hand while I was put to sleep.

I remember waking up in recovery and the nurses talking to me. I was somewhat nauseated and in a lot of pain. They gave me medication for both the nausea and pain. Dr. Geoffrey came to see me, and said that he had spoken to Jan, and that everything went well. Once the pain was under control, I could go home. It seemed like it was just minutes and the nurses were helping me get dressed and put me into a wheelchair. I was going home!

We got home and Jan helped me to bed and I went to sleep. Wayne got home and came into the bedroom to see me. I remember telling him that I was all right. He and Jan talked for quite some time in the kitchen. She made him something to eat, and then he called my sons. They both came into the bedroom and asked if I wanted some fruit to eat. Wayne helped me out of bed and Jan cut some fresh fruit. I don't recall any conversation, although they tell me I did talk, some of it not making much sense at all.

Jan came over the next morning, early, after Wayne had gone to work. I got up and we went out on the patio. She brought my favorite, Starbucks Chai Tea! I wasn't having much pain, but I was tired. We talked for a while. At this point, I wasn't thinking about the next surgery. I just wanted to get through this one. She told me that I was to see Dr. Leber in two days and that she would take me. She also told me that she and Wayne had a nice conversation. She knew that he was scared, but didn't tell him that I would be all right. She said that he needed to learn that for himself. She is an amazing social worker with a spiritual connection to the universe and all it's splendard.

I called my sons and I told them how I was doing, and that the surgery went well. I was walking and talking. They were concerned about the pain, but I told them that

I wasn't having much. Aaron and Evan were all right and glad to hear that I was doing well. Brady, well, he was still angry and didn't want to talk, but said that he was happy I was okay.

Jan took me to see Dr. Geoffrey; he said that everything went well and the incision looked good. He thought that I should wear the abdominal binder for comfort until the next surgery, which was scheduled for May 5th. Jan brought me home and said that if I needed anything to call her. I was just going to lie down and sleep, and wait for Wayne to come home.

The next two and a half weeks went by quickly and the anxiety of the next surgery was beginning to take its toll on me. But, I tried to maintain a positive attitude because I knew that if I didn't, Wayne would get more worried than he already was. If he didn't have something to worry about, he would find something. He didn't talk much about his concerns, or fears. He spent a lot of time at work because he was concerned about our finances. I tried to reassure him we would be all right. I needed him to be home with me.

Debbie Ziemann, RN

I went to see Dr. Geoffrey before the mastectomy, to sign the consents. This time, the surgery would last five hours and I would be in the hospital for three to five days. This time, I would have to have someone with me for a week when I went home from the hospital. Dr. Geoffrey said that he did not want me left alone at home without help. I wasn't sure what to do. I really could not ask people from work to take time off to spend the day with me. I told Wayne that I was going to call Aaron and see if he would come. We would pay for the airline ticket.

I called Aaron and I asked if he would be able to come and spend a week if we paid for the airline ticket. He would come. After finding out about the fraud, I called Aaron back and told him what had happened, and that we would not be able to get the ticket. I told him that I would be all right and would figure out something else and he said he would be here. In one hour, he called back and said that he was coming and that his father was paying for the ticket. He would fly in on Friday at 3:00 P.M. I told him that Wayne would pick him up, and that he should get his luggage and wait on the north side of the airport.

When I told Wayne that I wanted Aaron to come, he felt bad. He thought that I didn't think that he could take care of me. I asked him if he was going to take the entire week off and he said no. I reminded him that the doctor said that I could not be home alone for a week. I explained that Aaron could help me during the day and when he came home he could take care of me. I think then he understood, but was still felt hurt that Aaron was coming and that he himself would not be able to be at home with me.

Surgery was scheduled for ten in the morning. We had to be there at eight am.

There was little sleep the night before. We both tossed and turned, but didn't say anything to one another. We lay close, with our arms around each other, as if we were holding on for our lives. We were! This was to be the beginning of a long nine months. I didn't realize what I was going to go through emotionally and spiritually the next eleven months.

Nervously, we went to the hospital and registered. LouAnne came to sit with Wayne during the surgery. I didn't want him to sit there by himself. I asked her to make sure that he ate lunch. I was taken to a room to have the centennial biopsy done. They injected dye around the nipple and then took pictures. I was taken back to the holding area; Dr. Robert came to see us and said the

Debbie Ziemann, RN

pictures turned out good and there should be no problem with removing the node. Dr. Geoffrey came also. Today, he was quiet but still caring and compassionate.

The surgery took longer than expected, and I had problems after surgery, so they had to keep me longer in recovery. Wayne told me that I didn't get into my hospital room until after seven in the evening, and that he sent LouAnne home. He told me that her phone rang all day with people asking how I was doing. Dr. Robert came out and spoke to Wayne and LouAnne after the surgery, and told them that it went well. He was sure that they got all the cancer. The lymph node was soft and did not look like it had been invaded. The only thing that I remember that evening is that Wayne put my wedding rings on and said, "I love you."

The following day, Dr. Geoffrey came in to see me and took off the dressings. I remember him saying that he didn't like what he saw. I wanted to know what was happening, and he said the tissue was dying. I remember a sinking feeling in my stomach. He told me to start walking and asked about the pain. I told him that it was controlled with the morphine. I had a fever, and was drinking fluids, but had no appetite. I was to use a walker to walk and that I would have physical therapy to teach

38

SURVIVING BREAST CANCER

me how to get out of bed. I knew how to do that but I had no energy to tell him that. I didn't want to appear to be a "bad patient", as most nurses are.

Wayne came to the hospital and neither one of us had much to say. I was still hung over from the anesthesia and morphine, and he was tired and just didn't know what to say. I sent him home. I didn't sleep well that night. I could not understand why the tissue was dying, because I had not done anything that I wasn't supposed to. My heart was starting to fill with fear. Was I going to lose this breast that he had just made? Was I going to be left with just one breast, and if I did loose it, what could be done to make me whole again.

I had walked twice before Dr. Geoffrey came to see me, and he was pleased with that, but he was not pleased with the way the incisions looked on my abdomen and breast. I asked him if I could go home the next day and he said that he really wanted me to stay five days, but would see how I was tomorrow. I was disappointed. I just wanted to go home. I remember crying during the night. I wanted my husband to be with me. What had just happened to me, to us, was just starting to become real – I just lost my breast to cancer!

39

LouAnne, otherwise known as Precious, came to see me that day on her lunch. I showed her my new tummy (and the breast that you really couldn't see because of the dressing). It was good to see her. There was some laughing, and tears, because we talked about my fears and the cancer. The pathology report had not come back yet. Another restless night went by after Wayne and I talked and took a walk. I was walking better, standing straighter. He was quiet, showing concern, because he didn't want me to have any pain. We didn't talk about the mastectomy or the cancer. It was as if the word was a plague, that we were living twenty-thirty years ago, when you didn't talk about those things.

In the morning of the third day, Dr. Geoffrey called the nurse and asked if I still wanted to go home. She came in and asked me, and I told her that I did. She said that he would come see me before I went home. While I waited for Dr. Geoffrey, Diana came that day to see me. She was done seeing her patients. I told her I was being discharged and she offered to take me home. I called Wayne and told him that I would see him at home. Diana would go home after the surgeon came to get some things for me to use at home, a shower chair and walker.

SURVIVING BREAST CANCER

Dr. Geoffrey came and changed the dressings, wrote the prescriptions, and told me to see him on Tuesday. I asked if the pathology report was back. He said that it was and started reading it. It sounded so bad. I could feel the panic well up inside of me, tears starting to form in my eyes, Diana had gotten up, and stood by me, taking my hand. I had grown pale and tearful. Then Dr. Geoffrey stopped, and apologized. He said that normally he had his father do the reporting and reread the report. The margins of the tumor were clean; it was a Stage 2 with moderately rapid growth rate, and the centennial node was clean. I started to cry because that meant that it had not spread. I asked him if I could have a copy and he said that he would get one. He left and brought back a copy of the report. He went to write his progress note and write the prescriptions and came back in. He apologized several times and asked if I had read the report and if I was all right. I told him that I was okay.

Diana had left and came back to get me. We got the prescriptions filled and she stayed until Wayne got home. When Diana left our home, she told me that if we needed anything at all, to call. She would call me in the morning to see how I was doing. We hugged and said good-bye. I am not sure what I would have done without

41

LouAnne and Diana. They were a god-send. It was good to be home.

The first night in our own bed felt so good. Hospital beds are so hard and uncomfortable. There is too much noise in the hospital halls, and the peace and quiet of home was soothing. Wayne said that he was going to sleep in the other bedroom. I asked him why and he said that he didn't want to hurt me. I was hurt with the thought that he didn't want to sleep in the same bed with me. I asked if that was the real reason, or was it because he didn't want to lie next to me because I had my breast removed. Now, he was hurt, and told me that was not the reason, and, we did sleep in the same bed. We talked about our feelings, and I realized that he just didn't want to roll over and hit me, for fear he might hurt me. I told him that I was afraid that he would not want to touch me again because he would find me repulsive. I started to cry. He put his arms around me to console me, and reassured me that he loved me.

Friday was here and Wayne would be picking Aaron up at the airport on his way home from work. I was excited, but scared. I wasn't sure how Aaron would react. I didn't know if he would be able to help me with the dressings because he might be embarrassed seeing his mother's breast. I hadn't been dressed since I got home, sleeping in the afternoon. I was not having that much pain, just when I would get in and out of bed, or up from a chair. The abdomen and breast were both numb. I did have some muscle spasms in the abdominal area, but not many. I would sit outside for short periods because it was so hot, and looking at our pool made me angry because I could not get in and enjoy it. My mood was somewhat melancholy, not happy but not sad. I kept touching the breast, wondering if I would ever feel the same or if my life would ever be the same.

I heard the garage door open. I walked to the back door, and Aaron opened the door. The expression on his face said it all. He smiled, and there was a glow of relief that just filled his face. He said, "Hi Mama!" and held on to me as if there was no tomorrow. It felt good to have him in my arms. I held Wayne and kissed him hello. He still was uncomfortable with Aaron being here, but he understood why I wanted him here. I got dressed and we took Aaron to dinner and had a nice time. I fatigued really easy, so I went to bed and Wayne and Aaron stayed up for awhile and talked.

Wayne worked on Saturday, so Aaron and I just hung around. He cleaned the pool. When he was done, I asked if he wanted to see my breast, because he could not understand what had been done when I explained it to him. I felt some anxiety about doing this because I am his mother. And, I was afraid that he would be appalled at my appearance. I unbuttoned my top, and showed him the breast. To my relief, he was amazed at what the surgeon had done. We talked about implants and I told him that I wasn't going to have that done. Little did I know that eventually I would.

Aaron took me to see Dr. Geoffrey. There was no one in the waiting room. They called me in, and I asked Aaron if he wanted to go in with me. To my surprise, he did. I was again getting anxious. Dr. Geoffrey was going to remove the drain in the axilla area. He cut the stitches that were holding it in place and told me that it would be uncomfortable. Uncomfortable was not the word! I hollered and raised my hand and unfortunately smacked him in the face! I felt so bad. I was just trying to reach up to be able to squeeze his arm. I apologized numerous times, and he kept saying that it was okay. He finished and then put some pressure on the site so that it didn't hurt as much. Then he removed the drains from my abdomen. Those did not hurt much at all.

Walking out, I told Aaron that I felt so bad because I hit Dr. Geoffrey in the face. Aaron said that he didn't seem to mind and that he knew that it was an accident. Aaron told me that he almost left because he saw that it hurt so much when he took out the drain. I have never heard any of my sons say that they didn't like to see me hurt, whether physically or emotionally. I was deeply touched by his sensitivity.

The rest of the week, Aaron changed the abdominal and breast dressings during the day. I had shown Wayne how to do it so that he would feel better about taking care of me, and accept Aaron being here during the day better. His hands would shake when he changed the dressings. He didn't want to cause me any pain. Aaron was here for a week, and we did do some things together, but mostly stayed home and just talked. I would take a nap in the afternoon and then get up before Wayne came home from work and get dinner.

Aaron left early in the morning on Monday and I could drive. I didn't go anywhere, but it was nice to know that I could drive. LouAnne would call and come over. We would talk about different things. I was starting to have difficulty coping. The wounds were not healing and

I was to see the oncologist. Fear was starting to build up and I was even afraid to talk about it.

I sat in the oncologist's waiting room and my heart was pounding. I was nervous. I didn't know what he was going to say. The room was full, with people coming and going. They were there for chemotherapy. I became tearful seeing the women without hair. They were pale, and looked fatigued. Most of them did not smile. The spark in their eyes was gone. It was as if their life had been taken away from them: that they were just *existing*. I didn't want to be that way. I kept repeating to myself that Dr. Robert was very positive that I would just have to take Tamoxifen.

The oncologist came in the room and introduced himself. He sat in front of me on a stool. He went over the pathology report and then told me my treatment options. It was chemotherapy! Then, the Tamoxifen! My heart raced, and I felt like I had been hit in the chest. The drugs that he would give me were Cytoxin and Adriamycin.

I was familiar with these drugs. My mother had taken them. They made her nauseated; she would vomit for several hours, and she lost all her hair. I remember her sitting in a chair with hot flashes that you could see

SURVIVING BREAST CANCER

happening as her skin turned bright red around her neck and her face.

He told me that the decision was mine, but that he felt that chemotherapy was the best option. If the cancer came back, it would either go to the bone, lung, or liver, and that there was no cure. At fifty-two years old, with a new husband, I didn't think that I had much choice. I agreed to the chemotherapy. He wanted to know if I had any questions, but I was so disappointed that I could not think of any. My thought process went from curative to palliative, and this was not what I was expecting. I left, nearly running out of the building, and sat in my car for fifteen minutes trying not to cry, because I had to go see Dr. Geoffrey.

I was upset when I walked into Dr. Geoffrey's office, and Bonnie knew it by looking at me. She got me in right away. I told him that if I had known there was going to be so many problems I would not have had the TRAM flap done. I just would have had his Dad remove the breast. He said that he would not have done it if he did not think that it would work. He was perceptive; he knew that I was upset about something. He asked what had happened. So I told him that I had seen the oncologist, and what he has said. There was disappointment on his face. He felt so bad because they had told me I most likely would not need chemotherapy. I told him when my first treatment was. He said that it would slow the healing down. My heart sunk to my toes once again. He saw the tears running down my face. I told him that I didn't want any more surgery: no implants, no belly button, nothing! He told me not to think about that right now. I needed to remember that the chemotherapy was preventative. The cancer was gone, and that we had some minor set backs, but that he would see me through this. He held me and told me that he was here for me. I told him thank you, and he gave me so much comfort when he spoke to me, and let me tell him what I was feeling. He was appreciative of that comment and kissed my cheek.

Before the week was over, another problem occurred. I had dead fat tissue that opened the suture line during the night and there was blood and fat all over the bed. I was frantic! I called Bonnie in the office and she had me come in right away. I was crying and apologizing. He told me that it happens, and that it would be all right. I just could not understand what I had done wrong to have all this happen. I was getting more fatigued and crying more.

I had not energy to do anything. We have a beautiful back yard that we had worked so hard on, and I could

SURVIVING BREAST CANCER

not even take care of it. We have a pool; and I could not even go swimming. Wayne would not even get in the pool because he didn't want me to feel bad. We loved to get in the pool together, lounge on a raft, or play volleyball. All that had been taken away from me. I was angry that I could not swim. I didn't have the energy to clean the house and I just didn't want to do it anymore. Doing the laundry every week was a chore in itself. I felt that I was becoming a burden to my husband. I thought that he was avoiding me, because he was working such long hours. I started to think that he just didn't want to be married to me anymore because I was not the same person that he had married. I could not separate the person on the inside from the person on the outside.

Jan and I kept in touch by phone, and we would talk about all the problems that I was having. I would cry and just say that I wanted to get on with my life. A sense of urgency was taking over. I wanted to be able to do the things that I always wanted to do. I wanted to be able to put my hands into some rich, black soil, smell the freshly cut grass, sit in the shade of a tree, travel, and spend more time with Wayne and my sons. Priorities were changing. I would keep asking, "Why now? Why, when my life was just starting with Wayne?" I was going to bed at night after Wayne was asleep because I was afraid to have him see me. I was afraid that he would touch me and be displeased.

I felt like I was a sinking ship at sea.

At my next appointment with Dr. Geoffrey, he made a call to the oncologist, and postponed the chemotherapy. He let me talk about how I was feeling emotionally. He validated my feelings and gave me support. He hugged me before he left and said that he would get me through this again. He still had a couple tricks left up his sleeve.

I saw him every week, but after three weeks, he decided that he could close the wounds. This would mean another surgery. He said that they looked good and he didn't want to delay the chemotherapy much longer. Surgery was scheduled for the next week as outpatient.

It was now eight weeks since the first surgery. I asked Diana to go with me because the surgery would be outpatient. He was able to close both wounds. I remember, in the recovery room he came up to me and said that everything went well. I started to cry. He asked if I was in pain and I told him that they were tears of joy. He hugged me and told me to see him in two days. The nurses helped me dress and Diana took me home. I called

Wayne to let him know that I was home. Diana and I sat out on the patio and had a coke and talked. I wasn't in pain. My abdomen from numb from the previous surgery. We talked about how this entire event had changed our lives. That nothing would ever be the same.

I would always have a fear that it would come back; that I would be reminded of it, every day, when I changed clothes, got out of the shower. I told her it had been weeks since Wayne and I had been intimate. I was worried that he just didn't want to be with me anymore. She told me that he probably didn't want to burden me with that. He loved me, and he was going to be with me. She reminded me that there are other ways of showing affection: holding hands, kissing, and touching one another. She wanted to know if Wayne knew how I felt. I told her that I hadn't told him yet. She urged me to tell him. I told her that I was afraid, and she reminded me that he married me for who I am on the inside.

I was getting so depressed that I felt I needed to return to work. I thought that work would occupy my thoughts and make me feel better. And then it happened again! There were areas in the new abdominal incision that had opened. Nothing was healing right. There was another area on the breast that was draining, also. I called the office and went to see him that same day. He put a drain in. Two days after the drain was put in, I was taking a shower, and it fell out. It was after hours, and I paged Dr. Geoffrey and he called back. I told him what had happened and he said maybe it was trying to tell us something. He told me to pack it gently as before and come into the office the following day. I went to the office and he told me that he wanted to take me back to surgery and clean out those two areas that were not healing.

By this time, I had started chemotherapy again. I had already had one treatment. The surgery was scheduled for the end of the following week. I remember it was a Saturday before the surgery and my hair started falling out by the hand full. Wayne was at work; I sat on the couch and cried. I really needed him to be home. I went to the store and bought some bandanas, because I had decided that it would be better to just buzz it all off rather than watch it fall out in patches. So, when I got home from the store, I put a towel over the hand sink, and used Wayne's trimmer to shave my head.

I stood on front of the mirror and cried. I looked at the hair that was on the towel. It was white and gray. I stood looking in the mirror and thought how hideous I looked and how could Wayne think anything else. This was not the woman that he married! The tears continued to run down my face, my heart filled with fear and despair, I put some in a plastic bag and put it in my journal. I was sitting on the couch when Wayne got home, and he saw that I had been crying. I told him what had happened and what I had done. He wanted to see but I wouldn't let him. I am sure that made him feel bad but at the time, I just could not let him see me without any hair. I thought I looked hideous! An old bald lady; mutilated and deformed. How could Wayne not feel the same? I wanted to run away. But I couldn't. I needed him so much.

Jan had called me before the surgery, and I started crying when I told her that I had to have another surgery to clean the pocket in the breast. I was so tired of all the problems. I just wanted the wounds to heal so that I could get on with my life. The sense of urgency was growing and I couldn't control it. I had no energy to do anything. I was on the patio and she asked me to do something. She wanted me to go sit in the sun, close my eyes, and place my right hand just above the breast. She wanted me to concentrate on the color of white and purple. I told her I would. I went out by the waterfall and sat in a chair that was in the sun. I did some slow deep breathing to relax and closed my eyes. I placed my right hand just above my right breast and concentrated on the colors of

53

purple and white. I suddenly felt warm energy from my hand reaching into the breast. The breast was tingling with energy. I am not sure how long I sat there. I could feel myself relaxing and becoming peaceful. I knew that everything was going to be just fine.

When Wayne got home I told him what Jan had asked me to do, and how I felt the energy from my hand and the tingling in my breast. He was amazed. He could not believe what I was telling him. I was hoping that maybe, just maybe that this would take care of everything. But I could not help but have doubts.

Wayne took me to the surgicenter to have the pocket cleaned and the breast revised. The surgery was scheduled for 10:00 A.M. At 10:30 A.M., the nurse came out. She said that Dr. Geoffrey was running behind, because the surgery that he was doing was taking longer than expected. I sat, held Wayne's hand, and began to cry.

I had a cap on my head and I felt that everyone was looking at me. I felt so ashamed and embarrassed without hair; humiliated. The nurse came out again and said that it would be about noon before I would be having surgery. I asked if I could leave and come back. She said no. I told

SURVIVING BREAST CANCER

her that I couldn't wait. I was crying. I could not sit there any longer, feeling so self- conscious.

I was scared about what was going to happen when I got in there, because nothing had been going right. She went and told him. She then came out and said that Dr. Geoffrey wanted to talk to me. She took me back to a waiting area. He came in and asked me what was wrong. I told him that I just couldn't sit there any longer. I started crying and told him how I was feeling and that I was scared. He took off the dressing and probed the pocket and said that it was smaller, which meant that it was healing on its own. He said that if he had seen me in the holding area, he would probably have cancelled the surgery. I apologized for being such a baby and he asked me, "You haven't really cried yet, have you?" I told him no, and pointed at my head. I told him that I was embarrassed without any hair. He smiled and said, "You look good; look at me." I told him he looked good bald, but that I didn't. It wasn't normal. He held me and said that I was all right. He understood and that he would get me through this.

I was still crying on the way home. I told Wayne that I was sorry that I had him take the day off for nothing. He told me that I had nothing to apologize for. Then,

55

he reminded me what Jan had me do. He said that he never believed in things like that, but maybe, there was something to it. The wound was smaller than it was the day I saw Dr. Geoffrey in the office and he said that he would have cancelled the surgery anyway.

There is a connection between the body, the mind, and the soul. I realized that spending more time with positive thoughts and staying relaxed would help me heal physically. I have not been negative about this devastating event in our life. Every thought and feeling that I have had has been normal. It was just taking so long. What should have lasted two months was now in the third month.

I made my weekly visits again, and this time he came in and hugged me before he did anything at all. He asked how I was feeling. He thought that I looked better, and the wound was much smaller. I asked if I could go back to work. He wasn't real sure that I should. I told him that I thought I needed to, so that I didn't spend so much time home alone thinking. He gave me a release to go back to work. I would continue to have chemotherapy once a month and see him every two weeks. He thought it would be better for me emotionally to reduce the number of visits, but reinforced that if I needed to see him to call. I

SURVIVING BREAST CANCER

felt sad about not going every week. I wasn't ready to lose some of the most valuable support that I had had.

We hugged again, and I told him that I felt so much comfort when I talked to him. I didn't think that I could get through this ordeal with out his support. He always took the time to listen, asked the right questions to have me ventilate my feelings, and then validated those feelings with positive thoughts. I realized that of all the surgeons that I had to choose from, I was drawn to him and his father because I would need his strength, compassion and kindness to struggle through this. There are not many surgeons that would take the time to listen, who would emotionally support their patients.

I was anxious once again, because I thought I was going to lose the breast. The fat tissue kept dying! Then, what? Could he save it, or would he have to remove the breast? And then what he do? He came in and I showed him what had happened. I remembered that I started crying and he took my hand. I told him that I was afraid that I was going to lose the breast. He said that he hadn't seen anything like this other than in people who smoke He wasn't sure that he could save it, either, but he was not going to give up. I had to go back in one week.

When I went back, he said that he didn't need to take me back to surgery. I was so happy. I sat in my car, and just cried with tears of joy. Maybe things were starting to go the right way now.

It is October now, and the chemotherapy is over. I am fatigued, and I'm experiencing severe leg pain. I cannot sleep because of the pain. I've seen Dr. Geoffrey every two weeks, and now it is time to schedule the next surgery: the implants to make the breasts symmetrical. He discussed both types: saline and cellulose. I would have to be enrolled in a study for the cellulose implants. I chose the saline implants. He went over all the complications that could happen, but he knocked on wood and said, "Let's hope nothing happens." He wanted to wait three weeks, and I would have to stay overnight.

Surgery was early in the morning. Wayne and I were waiting in the holding area when he came. He smiled, but wasn't his usual self. He pulled the curtain around the gurney, and Wayne stepped outside. I didn't want him to leave, but I knew that he would not want to see Dr. Geoffrey taking pictures, or drawing on my breasts. I had to take off my gown and he measured my chest and drew with a marker. I was embarrassed and nervous, just like the first time. Uncontrollable tears ran down my face.

SURVIVING BREAST CANCER

I was afraid that there would be complications again. Dr. Geoffrey made me nervous for the first time, because he was not his usual self. He was quiet and didn't smile. It made me scared. I began to think that maybe he was not confident about doing the surgery this time. Lying on the surgical table, I was crying and Dr. Geoffrey came and took my hand. I held it tight. I was scared, really scared!

The surgery took longer than he had thought. He talked to Wayne and said that the surgery was very difficult. They sat down. He had to remove a lot of dead fat tissue. I remember in the recovery room, as he was standing beside me, he said that it was late, and he was going to have me admitted. I could go home in the morning. He made sure that I was not having much discomfort. I don't remember getting into a hospital bed, but I do remember the nurses coming and going.

In the morning, I cleaned up, and then went for a walk. Jan came shortly after and we walked around the halls waiting for Dr. Geoffrey. It was awhile before he came. He had been in surgery. He sat on the side of the bed and started to take off the dressings. He said they looked good. I started to cry: they were tears of joy. I was afraid that he was going to tell me that there was again some dead tissue. I had a drain and I had to measure the drainage and keep record of it. He gave me prescriptions and I was to see him in two days.

I went to the office on my next scheduled visit and it was time for the unveiling. He sat on a stool and I removed my gown. He face said it all. There was relief and pleasure. He told me that they looked good. They were healing well. He manipulated the implants and showed me how to do that. I was to do it twice a day. We discussed the last surgery: the nipple and belly button, and he wanted to wait six weeks, but wanted to see me before that. I told him that I was hoping to have it done before Christmas, and he said that he wanted to make sure that the breasts healed well. He promised that it would be done before New Year's Eve, so that I could begin 2005 with a new start.

He removed the drain and he was able to see the implant. That made him nervous. So he put in some sutures. He said that the tissue was thin from all the tissue that I had lost. He said that if it opened up and I could see the implant that I needed to come to the office right away. He would have to remove the implant and let it heal and then put another one in. If it opened and I couldn't see the implant, then he would re-close it and put me on antibiotics. As I left, I was concerned because it was one more thing that I had to worry about and be careful about.

I was getting anxious about the holidays when I went to see him. He was so pleased with the way things were looking. There is one thing about Dr. Geoffrey that I haven't mentioned, and maybe every plastic surgeon does this, but, he is forever taking pictures! Today was not any different! He got his camera. I told him that I was going to break that camera. He told me that it was to show him the progress following surgery, and he always looked at the previous pictures before I came in to see him so that he would be able to compare. He also used the pictures to help him determine what he needed to do for surgery. I told him that I understood that, but it just made me feel funny. We were talking and laughing and he told me that it was so good to see me smile and hear me laugh.

On December 30th, I had surgery for the nipple and belly button. This time it was done under sedation. I told him that if I started being unladylike, they better stuff my mouth with gauze! He just laughed and said that he didn't believe that I could *be* unladylike. I laughed and said, "You don't me very well."

Debbie Ziemann, RN

I didn't remember a thing. I don't even know if they had to put me to sleep. I did not ask either. I was in the recovery room and he told me that everything went great, and not to change any dressings. He wanted to see me in the morning at 9:00 A.M., and that I was to wait for him if he wasn't there. I hugged him and said, "Thank You. Please, don't take this wrong, but I love you." He said, "Thank you. It was not taken wrong." I was crying. He told me that 2005 would be a good year. We had made it through all this.

We went to the office the next day. It was New Year's Eve Day. Dr. Geoffrey took us into the exam room and he sat on the stool. He removed the dressings. Wayne was standing in the doorway, and he just stood there in awe. He kept repeating, "Look at that; it's amazing." A smile came across Dr. Geoffrey's face because he was happy that Wayne was happy. He said that the nipple looked good, and that it had good blood supply, and that the belly button would heal nicely. I was to go back on Tuesday.

Wayne has always been impressed with Dr. Geoffrey but having us come on the eve of the holiday even made him respect him even more, because his office was closed. He could not believe that he created something that he

SURVIVING BREAST CANCER

thought only God could do. We were lucky to have found such a wonderful surgeon.

I was driving to Dr. Geoffrey's office for my two-week follow up from surgery and I was thinking about the doctor-patient relationship coming to a close. I was feeling sad because a major part of my support system was coming to a close. Special people come and go in our lives, at times when we don't know why. I realized that I was drawn to these two surgeons, especially Dr. Geoffrey, because he would be the one that would give me the most strength. His kindness and compassion that he gave me made me feel good about myself. His positive attitude and compassion were what I had needed to get me through all that I was going through. I started to feel afraid that when I no longer needed to see him, that I would not be able to stay as strong and positive as I had been. Tears welled up in my eyes. He knew me better than most people, because he allowed me to express my feelings and concerns. He allowed me to cry, and gave me the emotional support that I needed at that moment.

He said that everything was healing well and that I didn't have to come back for a month. Tears started to run down my face. I told him what I had thought about on the way there, and he said that this was not good-bye. That if I needed to come and talk to him about life, I should call and come in. He understood how I felt. He hugged me and said that 2004 had been a long and difficult year, but that 2005 was going to be a good year!

I told him the oncologist had done some blood work because I could not tolerate the Tamoxifen and that I was going to go see him to discuss treatment options. To get me to talk more he said, "That is scary." I told him I was afraid, but I was sure that it would be to start another anti-estrogen medication because I had not had any scans done. He reaffirmed that he was just being thorough, and that he would keep me in is thoughts. He held me for a long time and told me that I was going to be all right, and that I was a survivor! He said that I am okay; I just have some bad days, and today was one of them.

I have seen death too often to
I Believe in Death.
It is not an ending – But a withdrawal as one
Who wishes to finish a Long Journey?
Stills the motor, Turns off the Lights,
Steps from his car and
Walks up the Path to the Home
That awaits him

_____John Blanding

Chapter Four
ANXIETY OF CHEMOTHERAPY

*D*riving to my first oncology appointment, I recalled Dr. Robert telling me that I would not need chemotherapy. I was holding onto those words. He was having me see an oncologist, just be too sure. But, something in my gut, as most nurses tend to believe, knew that I was going to have chemotherapy. His words were the bridge between what life had been and my life as it was now.

I signed in and completed a history and the insurance forms. The waiting area was divided into those for doctor appointments, and those for chemotherapy. I was frightened. I recalled my mother going through chemotherapy. It was difficult for her, and for my sister

Debbie Ziemann, RN

and me. Now, I was in the midst of it. Women came in with caps on their heads, because they had lost their hair. Their faces were gaunt, there skin dry, some were yellow in color, weak, or fatigued, and some reflecting hopelessness in their facial expressions.

My world, as I knew it to be safe, was shaken. I had been feeling helpless, out of control. My energy was out of balance. There is a sense of urgency to move forward. Now I am stuck in a place where I could not see clearly, could not appreciate the present moment. I was seeking meaning and purpose to my life and it was clouded, with no light for me to see the path.

I sat there, for what seemed to be hours. He finally knocked and entered. He was taking an in-depth history and then suddenly, he asked if I was a nurse. I responded yes, and told him that I worked for Hospice of Arizona. He said that he thought I was a nurse by my answers. He then completed a physical.

I got dressed and he returned in about fifteen minutes. He sat directly in front of me on a stool. He discussed the pathology report; it was an estrogen receptive tumor. He also said that the lymph nodes were not involved. He told me that the course of treatment could be Tamoxifen and chemotherapy: Adriamycin and Cytoxin were the two drugs that would be used. He said that if the cancer were to come back it would be in the bone, the lung, and or the liver, and as a nurse, I knew there was no cure. Although, I appreciated the honesty, it was something that I did not want to think about right then. I didn't want to hear that I could need to make a decision to be going through this once again in several years.

Reinforcing that the treatment was my choice, he advised chemotherapy. I put my head down, tears running down my cheeks. The silence was deafening. Then, he said the cancer was found fairly early. I looked up and told him about my mother going through chemotherapy and the complications that she had had from it. He told me that now there are medications they give prior to the treatment to prevent nausea and vomiting. Neupogen is given when the white cell count drops too low. I had to ask him, "If I was your family member, what option would you advise me to have?" The answer was chemotherapy. Through tears I told him I would take his advice.

The nurse came in with a booklet and papers. She said that I would lose my hair within seven to ten days of the first treatment, and possibly my eyebrows and lashes. My nails would not grow. She suggested that I use a non-alcohol based mouthwash and a soft toothbrush because my gums could bleed and I could develop sores in my mouth. I was to drink a lot of water and take my temperature every morning. After each treatment, my urine would be red. If I had any problems, or any other signs of infection, I was to call the office and speak to the triage nurse. I could call any time with questions and or concerns. I thought that he seemed to be receptive to the needs of someone in my position and showed concern. Later, I would decide not to see him anymore but find another oncologist.

When I left the office, and walked to the car, I started crying. I sat in my car for a while and asked my mother to share her strength and courage with me. I really needed her to be with me. As I sat there, collecting myself, my eyes were closed and I was thinking of a place far away, that was peaceful and beautiful. My mother appeared and sat down beside me. She took my hand and smiled and told me that I was going to be just fine. She touched my cheek and then got up and left.

I was told once that when something has happened in your life that is devastating, someone that you have lost, that you loved, will come to you and give you comfort. I never truly was sure that I believed that, but at that moment, I did. My mother was with me, watching over me. And she would help with this struggle.

I knew that when I returned home, I would have to be strong. No crying tonight because I had to tell my husband. Wayne is a Marine. You know the saying, "Once a Marine, always a Marine." Most of the time, he wears that marine hat, but when it come to me suffering, or having pain, or being hurt, that hat comes off and he is a six-foot-two inch Teddy Bear. I knew that when I told him, fear would well up inside his chest, his stomach would ache, and his hands would shake. I would have to make sure that he understood that it was preventative. I would also have to tell my sons.

Wayne did all right with the news. But, then he didn't express any anxiety. I remember sitting on the couch later beside him and he held my hand. I am sure that he felt that he was going to lose me. I told him that there would be some things that we would have to get before I started the therapy. I was feeling really low and I lay beside him as he held me. We went to bed that evening in silence. I lay facing him with my arm around his belly.

I was afraid when I went for my first treatment. The room had chairs along three walls, with intravenous poles and pumps at each chair. The nurse made idle chatter, which didn't make me feel any better. In fact, I was surprised. I thought they would ask questions that would allow me to talk about how I was feeling. They started the treatment and then left. I watched the activity in the room and realized that it was just an assembly line. The nurses were not talking to any one. There was no television, no headsets for CD players, magazines, or books. I was surprised that there was not a social worker. I was miserable. I became tearful. It was all right to cry and be scared, but I wanted someone to listen to what I was feeling.

I eventually had to have injections of the Neupogen. The oncologist told me that I would have some mild joint pain. I was not looking forward to that because I knew that it would be more than mild. I have osteoarthritis and had joint pain most of the time. I was not expecting the amount of pain that I did have. I could not sleep because of the pain in my joints and my bones. I hurt constantly. It even hurt to sit. On top of all that were the hot flashes and night sweats. The chemotherapy was destroying my ovaries so they would not produce estrogen. The positive of that was that I knew it was working. Then, I developed some muscle weakness and the pain got worse. I called the office and left a message that I was having problems

SURVIVING BREAST CANCER

and what they were. The nurse called me back and told me that the doctor wanted me to go to the emergency room.

I was not happy about that, but I understood why. He was going to have them do a bone scan to see if the cancer had already spread. In my heart, I knew that what he wanted was right, but I didn't want to hear it. I knew that these symptoms were from the Neupogen. I didn't go to the emergency room. I called them on Monday and the nurse called me back and talked to me about how I was feeling. I told her and she told me to try Advil at bedtime. I was to let them know if I had any other problems.

I was losing confidence in the oncologist. Not because he was not good at what he does, but because he was distant, and seemed uninterested in what I was feeling emotionally and spiritually. He never asked how I was doing. His exams seemed superficial: done because he had to, not because he was interested in if there was something else going on.

The fourth treatment had to be cancelled because my white cell count was too low. I started to get teary and he handed me a Kleenex. I told him that would postpone the last surgery. He said that as a nurse, I knew that he could not give me the treatment because it was too risky. That made me angry. I told him that as a nurse I understood that, but that I was not a nurse right now: I was a *human being* who had been diagnosed with breast cancer, had a mastectomy, and now chemotherapy. Being a nurse did not negate any feelings that anyone else had in this situation. I was still dealing with a loss, and going through the grieving process. I just wanted to get through this part of the process so that I could go on with the rest. He did not respond.

As I was getting closer to the end of the treatments and surgery, I made two calendars: one, for the countdown to the last treatment, and the other for the last surgery. When the last treatment was postponed, I tore the calendars up. I realized that they did not allow me to be flexible. I am such a structured person and I set deadlines. I was setting expectations of my body that it could not meet.

I was once again feeling that my path to recovery was clouded; there was no light at the end of the tunnel. I did not know who I was and where I was going. I was confused and disgusted with the way that I looked. I had to wear a wig because I didn't want anyone to see me without hair. I could not stand to look at the reconstructed breast. I was so ashamed of how I looked, that I found myself avoiding my husband. I would stay up later than he did till I knew that he was asleep and then go to bed. I didn't want him to touch me or see me without hair.

When I realized what I was doing I told him. He was getting ready for work one morning and I apologized for what I had been doing to him. I was crying when I told him, and he held me and told me that he loved me for who I was on the inside. It didn't matter if I had one breast or two, if I had hair or not. It didn't change who I was. He married me for the person that I am. He told me that we would get through this together. I was stuck with him for the long haul. I felt some relief with his words. Holding me gave me such comfort. He asked what I had said to him on our wedding day.

I told him that I had said, "You loved me for who I was, and for who I am now, and you love me for who I will become." He told me that I needed to remember that because he would love me forever.

The chemotherapy was now complete. I would start the Tamoxifen. Once again I was told that I would have some mild breastbone and hip pain. Once again, they were wrong. It was close to Thanksgiving. I was unable to sleep because of the pain. I had a difficult time driving because my hips, knees, ankles, and legs hurt so badly. I had not experienced the muscle pain before. I had problems with my vision: my eyes would get tired and I could not see very well. But, the worst was that I was crying all the time. I would wake in the middle of the night. I was crying at work and was putting my job in jeopardy. I did not want to be at work. I was overwhelmed with everything. The upcoming holidays were making me so anxious. I wanted to run away, dig a hole, jump in and hide till it was all over. As much as I wanted and loved Wayne, I wanted him to go. As much as I wanted to see my sons at Christmas, I didn't want them to come.

I called the optometrist and made an appointment to have my eyes checked. I just had my eyes examined in March, but I could not see very well up close or far away. I called the oncologist and talked to the nurse. She called me back and told me that he wanted me to have my eyes checked, and to hold the Tamoxifen for three weeks. I was to call back which would have made it the week of Christmas and let him know how I felt.

My eye exam showed minimal changes, so I didn't need a new prescription. By then end of the three weeks, I was feeling better. I still had the muscle pain but not the severe bone pain. I was no longer crying all the time.

SURVIVING BREAST CANCER

I knew that life would never be the same and I realized that I was struggling to find a new identity. I was still anxious about Christmas with my sons. How would they react when they saw me? What would they think about my wig? Would I need to be careful not to walk out of the bedroom without it?

I called the week of December 20th, and told the oncologist nurse that I was feeling much better, the crying had stopped, the bone pain was much better, and my vision was now back to normal. I asked about a new medication for breast cancer call Arimidex. She said that she would talk to him and get back to me.

When she did call, she said that the Arimidex was for post-menopausal women and he wanted to know if I was. I told her that I only had my ovaries and I did not know. So he wanted some lab work done. By the end of the week, the doctor himself called me and said that the blood work showed that I was peri-menopausal. He wanted to discuss treatment options with me, but wanted me to come into the office next week. He did not want to talk to me on the phone. So I made an appointment for the following week.

Debbie Ziemann, RN

I was hesitant to go. I remembered all the feelings that I had sitting in the waiting area. I had to sit there for forty-five minutes before they called my name. I paged LouAnne because I was so anxious and afraid of what he might say. I thought of all the things that he could possibly tell me: more chemotherapy; having another surgery to remove my ovaries; another oral medication; or nothing at all. She paged me back and said that it was all right to be nervous. She would be, too. I should let myself be anxious. It was okay! And just have a miserable day if that is what it took.

I was taken back to a room. I had to wait there for another thirty minutes.

When he came in he sat in front of me on a stool and repeated what he had told me on the phone. He thought that the Arimidex would be appropriate for me to take because I would be going into menopause rather quickly. He had had a lot of success with this medication and there were very few side effects. Probably the most I would have would be some mild joint pain, and that it could cause osteoporosis. I told him that I had looked the medication up on the Internet and found that it had all the same side effects as Tamoxifen. I never had mild bone pain; it was moderate to severe. He said that only three percent of the

SURVIVING BREAST CANCER

people have not been able to tolerate the medication. I agreed to try and he told me that if I could not tolerate it we would stop it.

He started to get up, and I told him that I had some questions, so he sat back down. I wanted to know what other treatment there would be if this didn't work and he said let's see what happens first. He obviously didn't want to spend any more time with me or answer my questions because he started to get up again. I told him that I still had a couple of more questions.

I had gone there with a list so I had to quickly prioritize them. I wanted to know what tests would be done for follow up, because none had been done. He just responded that I would need blood work in four months and to see him. The last question was difficult for me to ask because I don't talk about my bedroom life. I told him that I knew there could be nothing done for my libido. My heart wanted to be intimate with my husband but my body did not want to respond. His answer was to see a gynecologist and he got up and left saying that a nurse would bring me the lab slip and a prescription. The nurse also said that he suggested that I have my ovaries removed. WOW!

He didn't even mention that when he was with me and now, he suggested it.

I sat there feeling let down. He did not want to spend time with me and answer my questions. There I was; someone who had just been diagnosed with breast cancer, had a mastectomy, and went through chemotherapy, and he didn't want to take the time to answer my questions! This was an oncologist who got into this business to help people through difficult times, people whose emotions are like a roller coaster, needing to have time spent with them, to have questions answered no matter how silly they may be to him, and be emotionally supported.

I became angry and before I had left the office, I had decided that I was not going back to him. He was fired! I don't want my hand held, but I do expect to be treated as a person and be able to have questions answered! I wanted to know what other tests would be done to ensure that the cancer had not spread already and to ensure that if it did come back, that it was found quickly. I wanted to know if I would ever be able to respond to my husband physically and have a satisfying sex life.

I continued to have the muscle pain and sought the advice of the nurse practitioner that I have been seeing for three years. Once I described the pain that I was having, she said that I had fibromyalgia. I was not surprised. I have had chronic fatigue for several years.

Fibromyalgia is very common in women who have breast cancer and have gone through chemotherapy. It is an autoimmune disorder. She gave me a prescription for a mild muscle relaxant and told me to have massages. I told her that we bought a hot tub and she thought that would be very beneficial too.

The muscle relaxant was working. I had minimal discomfort. I had a massage without any residual muscle pain, and I was able to sleep through the entire night without waking in pain. I started the Arimidex and after four days, I have now started having bone, joint, and back pain. I was having difficulty sitting for long periods of time and when I got up, my legs and hips were very uncomfortable. I had now decided that I would have my ovaries removed and continue the Arimidex until I saw the new oncologist.

Dr. Robert Leber referred me to a gynecologist. As a general surgeon, he was no longer permitted to remove ovaries. So, I made an appointment. Sitting in the gynecologist's waiting room, I was very anxious. I had to wait for what seemed to be lifetime. Tears formed in my eyes because I knew that he was going to be in agreement to have my ovaries removed.

All I could think about was that I would be having another surgery and what if, this time they found more cancer? What would happen then? What path would that take me on? I didn't know if I would be strong enough, and even willing to go through more chemotherapy.

I had nearly stopped before the first course of chemotherapy was done. I had been so fatigued and suffered severe bone pain. I remember that my husband came home from work one evening and I was in tears. I told him that I didn't know if I could finish the treatments.

He held me and told me that he understood. I told him that I had only agreed to the chemotherapy because of him and my sons. I know that he didn't understand. He was holding me so tightly I could feel him tremble with fear. I knew that he was afraid that he would lose me to this cancer, just as our life had started together.

I could feel the depth of his love and devotion when he held me. I started to relax and I told him that I would continue, completing the course of treatment. I

SURVIVING BREAST CANCER

let him know, however, that I didn't know that, if the cancer came back, if I would be able to go through the chemotherapy again. Sometimes the treatment is worse than the disease!

To my surprise, the gynecologist himself came to the waiting area and called my name. He introduced himself and took me to his office. He did a detailed history. He told me that he was in agreement with the other physicians; that I should have my ovaries removed. I would be in the hospital for two days and the recovery normally was five to six weeks.

I was taken to another room and given a gown for a breast and pelvic exam. I was shaking inside. I was afraid of what his reaction would be when he saw the reconstructed breast and the scar on my abdomen. I raised my arms above my head for the breast exam, and as he opened the gown to examine the breasts, his facial expression revealed what I had feared: He looked mortified! He was afraid to touch either breast! He looked at my abdomen after he had completed the pelvic exam and looked at the scar and said that it didn't look good, but he could make the incision in the scar.

Debbie Ziemann, RN

Fear just overwhelmed me. I was afraid to have the surgery: Reopening the scar from the last surgery that healed so poorly, and I had wounds that took forever to heal. I was scared that would happen again.

Tears ran down my face. I knew that it was all right to cry and be afraid. I told myself that I had to "suck it up," stay in control. I didn't know this doctor and I didn't know what he would think or feel about me crying or being afraid.

I went to the front desk and the nurse gave me a lab slip and informed me that she would schedule the surgery. I told her that it couldn't be done till the last two weeks of March. My husband was having surgery on March first.

After seeing the gynecologist, I immediately called Dr. Geoffrey. I explained what the surgeon had said, and his concerns about the abdominal scar, and asked if he would assist the gynecologist. He said that he would be happy to. I was to ask him to call Dr. Geoffrey and that the nurse should call Bonnie and coordinate the surgery with both their schedules.

I received a call three days later, and the surgery was scheduled for the 22nd of March and Dr. Geoffrey would

SURVIVING BREAST CANCER

assist. A sense of relief filled my heart, and I was less concerned about the surgery. I thought about Dr. Geoffrey and how much I missed seeing him. I needed the strength that he gave to me when I was anxious and afraid.

The pressure at work had been horrendous! I had to tell my supervisor about the upcoming surgery and how long I would be off. I was also afraid that I would not be able to return to the management position that I had. Having all these doctor appointments had put me in an awkward position. I felt I was being monitored closely, which made me feel uncomfortable and uneasy.

I was told that I would have to request a medical leave of absence from the administrator, and that I may not be able to have my team back. I also would have to pay Cobra if I was off that long. I looked at the calendar and decided that I would only take two weeks off after the surgery, because financially, we could not pay for Cobra. I requested the medical leave and spoke with administrator and informed her that I would be back in two weeks. The surgeon didn't know this yet, but I thought once I had explained why, and that I didn't do any lifting, that it would be all right.

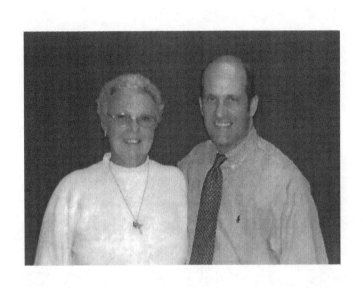

Chapter Five
AFTER THE TREATMENT, THE STRUGGLE BEGINS

"Personal suffering is a harsh, but grand teacher. Grief, like history, is a living process altered by how we navigate through the experience. It is also our way of letting go of life, as we knew it and embracing life, as it will grow to be. When we experience a break in our emotional, spiritual or physical connection, we naturally seek a new balance to restore control and harmony in life. As we accept our continued existence, our grief experience helps us find new ways, and perhaps incorporates old ways, to create new identity." (*Living Beyond Breast Cancer*; Marisa C. Weiss, MD and Ellen Weiss)

Debbie Ziemann, RN

The struggle really begins once the treatments are done. My body image had changed and I had difficulty accepting the way that I looked. I had no hair and I was afraid the wig that I was wearing didn't look real. How strange it was to place that thing on my head and try to comb it so that it looked like my hair. When strangers looked at me, I thought that they knew. If I wore a cap instead, some of the nurses said that it made them realize just how sick I was. I didn't want anyone to know. I did not want to be set apart from others.

I could not look at myself in the mirror. I had one normal-looking breast for my age, and the other was larger, and covered with dressings. I didn't want my husband to touch me. I even thought that if he did, he would think that I was grotesque. He didn't reach out to touch me to have intimacy. I began to think that he didn't want to be with me anymore, or that maybe he did find me to be gross (for a lack of a better word). At the same time, I wanted to be with my husband, even though I had no desire to have sex. I knew that the chemotherapy had destroyed my libido.

I thought that once the treatments were over I would be able to do the things that I enjoyed doing. But I had no energy. The breast cancer experience is itself enough to

86

drain all energy from the toughest woman, I think. I had thought I was a pretty tough person. There is uncertainty from the moment you think you have something to worry about, to the initial doctor visit when the diagnosis of breast cancer is laid on you, to the waiting of all the test results. And, there are the questions, followed by answers and more questions.

The fear and anxiety of recurrence never leaves. It is like you are hanging your life out on a clothesline and watching it dry out! I found that those things that I did enjoy nine months before were no longer a priority. It took everything that I had to work a full day. I would come home and just cry because I was lost! I didn't know who I was or where I was going in life.

I felt so bad for Wayne because he had to go through this with me. And, he was being so strong. He never cried (that I knew of). He would come home after a long day of work, take a shower, eat, and then watch television, falling to sleep in the chair. I would go to bed alone. Unknowingly to him, I would wake when he came to bed and lay there, silent, and wait for him to put his arm around me or touch me. It didn't ever happen. Tears would run down my cheek. I was afraid myself to reach out to him. What a web that I weaved; and I had no understanding of how to control it. I was out of control. There was no balance in my life.

I sought out a support group, hoping that the interaction with others that have been in my position would help me find who I was and where I was going. Sometimes, knowing that others have the same problems or feelings is helpful. There is validation of mutual feelings and emotions. But it didn't work; I found that the nurse in me took on their problems, and I was not able to deal with my own. I had to find another means to learn who I was and how to accept myself for the way that I looked now.

I started to write in my journal, every day, in the hopes that this healing ritual would help me move through the grieving process. As I went back and read some of it, I found that I had gone through all the stages of grief at different times along the way, through the months that seemed to have flown by. I even repeated some of the steps. I found that talking to Diana and LouAnne was the most helpful. They would remind me of what I would say to my patients. They validated my feelings and gave me hope. They reminded me that it was normal and all right to feel the way that I did: lost, anxious, and out of control. They reminded me that I was expecting too much of myself by setting expectations that my body could not meet which caused disappointment and frustration.

I wasn't allowing myself to be flexible, which ultimately caused me to lose confidence in myself. They were my support group; helping to restore the confidence that the diagnosis of cancer had shattered, to reclaim the control of my life that the cancer had stolen. They drew me into a community of understanding people who allowed me to connect, to share the good and the bad, and simply recover. They allowed me to share my journey with them.

I had to find a new, normal life. I didn't know what to do with myself. It was like I was in limbo. Cancer was still on my mind twenty-four hours a day. I felt very old. I thought that I looked very old, lost, looking into my grave. When you have been discharged, there is a corner in your mind reserved for "Cancer Worry." Every time something hurt or I got sick, I think that it is back. You're discharged, and you feel like you have been dumped. I felt more scared after the treatment was done than when it had first been diagnosed. There was a scheduled routine and a plan of attack, which were comforting...and now they were gone.

My friends and co-workers concluded that the disease was beaten and done with; they congratulated me, and celebrated with enthusiasm. I dreaded going to my own end-of-treatment party. I expected to feel great and back to normal and ready to get on with my life, but instead, I found that life would never be the same. I felt lost, in nowhere land, with the fear that the cancer would be back.

Then, I worried, "Did the treatment really work?" Separation anxiety takes on a new meaning. Some people who I work with expected me to be happy and to be in control of my emotions. There was one nurse in particular who was relieved when I was done with therapy and looked for me to be my old self: as if I could flip a switch and not be a cancer patient anymore – as if that were possible.

I thought I was dealing with the circumstances just fine, but I wasn't: I would have some really bad days at work. To make things worse, I had to pretend that I wasn't having a bad day. I realized that was not emotionally healthy. I would have bad days and it was okay to cry. It was all part of the healing process. It is part of the process of becoming a survivor!

I wanted to take better care of myself. I didn't want to waste time worrying about unimportant details. I wanted to take the time to "smell the roses." I wanted to enjoy things that I hadn't done or seen before. I wanted to start doing the things I had always enjoyed and now were just lost in a person of the past. I wasn't going to take anything for granted. I didn't want to waste time. I found, through writing in my journal, that I wanted to find new meaning from, and derive fulfillment from each moment of every day. I wanted to build memories.

Laughter and merriment are prized. Hugging now takes on a new importance. Taking care of myself had to be a priority. Realizing that if I felt like crying – then I should cry. I realized the biggest gift that I could give to myself was time – time for recovery. I could not allow anyone to make me feel guilty or take on something that I was not ready for.

Expectations had to be realistic for me, not anyone else. I had to learn that I am who I am; that disease does not define me. I will be able to get up in the morning and not have cancer be the first thought that comes to mind. I will be able to look in the mirror and not be ashamed of how I appear. My hair will grow back; maybe it will be a different color and texture, but it will grow back, and I

Debbie Ziemann, RN

will no longer need to wear that mop on my head. I had to take control of my life!

I didn't choose this disease. I had a good life before cancer, and there was no reason why it would not be good again. I had to learn that I had to live one moment at a time, one day at a time. I could not let the fear of cancer run my life. I would have a new life defined by what I wanted it to be.

Sometimes the Truth

That we are not alone is
a Rope that keeps us from Slipping,
much as the rope a climber clings to on the
Side of a mountain.

_____*Author Unknown*

Chapter Six
STATE OF MIND

Being a victim is a state of mind created by others,
A Survivor dictates their own state of mind!
A victim fears the moments of Grief,
A Survivor welcomes those moments!

A victim knows about feeling down and tries to stay up,
A Survivor knows that feeling down is Okay!
A victim tries hard to hide the tears,
A Survivor never leaves home without Kleenex!

A victim struggles to maintain a state of normalcy,
A Survivor knows normal no longer exists!
A victim gets caught in isolation,
A Survivor reaches out when they need to!

A victim sometimes feels guilty laughing,
A Survivor laughs through the tears!
A victim tries at times to block out the memories,
A Survivor embraces memories of all kinds!

A victim wants someone to cure their Grief,
A Survivor just wants someone to share their journey!
A victim struggles to get over the grief,
A Survivor fights to get through it!

A victim tries to get on with their life,
A Survivor lives their life knowing nothing will ever be
the same
A victim says "Oh, I'm okay...then secretly cries,
A Survivor openly cries...and says I'm Okay!"

_____*Author Unknown*

*B*eing a victim of the disease is a state of mind created by others; they do not want to share your journey with you. Once the treatment is over, society expects that everything should go back to normal. You are forced to hide your grief and fears. Therefore, you try and stay up when you feel down. You hide your tears and try to maintain a sense of normalcy. This attitude places you in isolation. A victim becomes afraid that they will forget everything. A victim will feel guilty for laughing, because it will block out the memories of what took place. A victim will struggle through their grieving process and want someone else to cure that grief.

There were a couple of nurses where I worked who tried to make me a victim. It was during the holidays, when I was having so much trouble with my mood. I was overwhelmed with preparing for a Christmas party that my husband wanted to have. He wanted to have all this food that I was to make. He wanted to invite staff from his workplace and mine, totaling about seventy-five people. I was not in the Christmas mood. I always loved Christmas. I would decorate every room in the house. It is a time when I could create a fantasy world and not have to worry about being hauled away! I did not know how I was going to get through this. I was crying all the time.

I understood why he wanted to have the party. It was tradition in his mother's home, and I believe that he was looking for some normalcy. He made the invitations and planned the menu. I would cry every time he talked about it. One day, he said that he knew that I thought it was overwhelming but he would help me. I told him that it wasn't a thought, I was overwhelmed and I didn't think that I could do it!

I didn't want to go to work in November and December. I would wake in the morning just overwhelmed with the thought of a party and my sons coming home for the holidays. I would talk to my co-workers about how I was feeling and just cry, sometimes just sob. I knew that nothing would ever be the same. Not work, not my family, nor my relationship with my husband. It was not

Debbie Ziemann, RN

that we had grown apart. We had grown closer than I ever thought possible.

One of the nurses told me that she thought I dwelled on the negative too much. I could not understand that. She thought that I should be happy. The cancer was gone, and I had another chance at life. I told her that losing a breast is far more complicated than she realized. That it was a loss, and that there is a process of grieving that goes with that. Our breasts are part of what society looks at that makes us female, they are part of our sexuality and our appearance. The emotions and feelings that I was experiencing were not negative. They were fact!

It was not possible for her to understand until she herself had to go through what I had gone through. Another nurse told me that all the crying had to stop. I was not to talk to my co-workers because I was placing a burden on them: they had their own personal problems. I was taking them away from their work. I was to pretend to be having a good day when I was having a bad day! I couldn't believe that! We are nurses and hospice nurses! If I could not cry at work and talk to them and be supported, why were we in the business of hospice?

I talked to Diana and Irene one day, when I thought that I was losing total control. They both told me that it was okay to cry. I was still grieving, and I needed to allow myself time to heal. That it was normal to know that the holidays would never be the same. I wanted my sons to come, but at the same time I didn't. I had always been their pillar of strength. They had never seen me cry or so lost and disoriented. Now the roles were changing. I was not comfortable with that. Diana held me and told me that my sons needed to feel their own pain. I could not feel it for them. She reassured me that my sons loved me for the person that I am inside, not how I look on the outside. The three of us cried together.

I did get through the holidays.

I was off the Tamoxifen, and in three weeks I was much better. The crying had stopped and I no longer was feeling like I was drowning in sorrow. I decorated the house, had a good time at our first Christmas party, and enjoyed my sons. They hugged me every time they saw me and told me they were glad that I was feeling better. At Christmas dinner, I said a blessing, thanking God for this difficult time, giving us strength to get through it, and bringing us closer together. My sons all said that they

Debbie Ziemann, RN

were glad that I was here for the holiday. I then knew the depth of their concern and fear.

There are several important steps that need to be taken to change that state of mind from victim to survivor. I needed to evaluate if hospice was the nursing career that I would be able to function in effectively. With facing my own mortality, knowing what patients feel like when they are told they have cancer, I know that I will be a better hospice nurse. The decision that I have to make though is, am I able to provide the support and direction while I am grieving and healing myself?

I had to re-evaluate my health care team. Trust and respect are the key elements to a good doctor-patient relationship. I want a doctor who loves his profession – because I know then he is doing all he can to be the best doctor for me. The personal qualities are just as important. They need to listen and take time with you. Listening is essential in a good doctor-patient relationship; a doctor who listens respects you. They need to be supportive, not having one foot in the door, showing that they are too busy to talk to you, to answer your questions, and to be supportive. They, in turn, need to ask questions, the questions that will allow you to tell them how you're feeling, about your spouse, and about your family.

There needs to be an optimistic attitude and body language that transmits the belief that you will live a long life. If there are complications with reconstructive surgery as I had, then that positive attitude is even more vital: to know that he was not giving up. They need to promoted a sense of teamwork. It seemed that no matter if I was having a good day or a bad day, when I left Dr. Geoffrey's office I felt better because he took the time to listen, asked questions, and gave me a lot of emotional support. He never gave up on me. He said that he would get me through the complications of the surgery. He was always honest with me; he never kept anything back. If he worried about something that was not healing right, or the way he thought it should have, he told me.

He didn't take away my sense of privacy, even when he took pictures, which it seemed happened on every visit. He knew that it made me uncomfortable, but he did it quickly, and then helped me get my gown back on. He never made me feel embarrassed. Dr. Geoffrey always knew when I was afraid. There was a connection, a bond that developed.

He would come in the room smiling and give me a hug. There was so much comfort I received from him. I was able to cry, laugh, and even be angry. I mention

Dr. Geoffrey by name because he has played such an important part of my recovery, of my Survival! He was not going to allow me to be a victim. I was going to be one of the Survivors!

Keeping in touch with your primary physician is important as well. The same qualities need to be present. I have been blessed with a family nurse practitioner who allowed me to cry, and express my concerns, and who really listened to what I was saying. She knew that if I was having a problem, or there were new symptoms that I was having, that they were real and she treated them. She has stood by me. She told me to call her at any time. She gave me her personal office number and her cell phone number. She always smiled and hugged me. I kept her informed of all the problems, the treatments, medications that had been prescribed, and any changes in medications and surgeries. I knew that eventually she would be the one doing all the follow up.

On my last visit to the oncologist, I realized that there was no connection. His foot was always in the door, not wanting to spend time with me to answer my questions, or give support. I had been going to him for several months feeling badly, and I always left feeling worse! I did not want him to hold my hand, but I was made to feel that

SURVIVING BREAST CANCER

I was not important to him as a person. Maybe that is a characteristic of oncologists. However, I don't want to stereotype them. I spent so much emotional energy investing myself in this relationship. It was hard to come to the decision that I needed to change oncologists, when I identified that there was a meaningful problem that was not going to go away.

I did some searching and found another oncologist who is absolutely wonderful. He smiles, asks important questions with sincerity, and gives me honest answers. He has made it easy to ask personal questions regarding my longing to have intimacy with my husband while having no desire or the ability to respond. He gave suggestions on how to improve that ability. He did tests to see why I was not able to respond physically. He informed me right at the beginning how often I would be seeing him, and when the time came to lessen the number of visits, he told me that we would reevaluate the timeline. He told me that after five years of close follow-ups, if it had caused too much anxiety, we could continue, so that I would have the reassurance that I needed until I was ready to make yearly visits. He loves his profession!

He also told me that he wanted to have genetic testing and counseling done. When they called me, I had to

101

complete a family history in detail. This included all family members on my paternal and maternal side of the family who had died from cancer. She would then schedule an appointment, which would take two hours. There would be lab work that needed to be done, and the results of those tests would take a month to come back. Then I would have to go back, and the results of those tests would determine what course of action would be taken.

Fear of the unknown started to build up in me and I started to cry. There is a history of cancer on both sides of my family. Every "what if?" came to my mind. What will the course of action be? Anxiety started to build up; my stomach felt like it had reached my toes! I called my husband and told him. I asked if he would be able to go with me for the first appointment. He told me that he would most definitely go! I didn't want to go alone. I needed his support and his strength. I was afraid that the cancer would come back in the other breast, or that I would be prone to lung, bone, or liver cancer.

I wasn't sure that I wanted to know all the information, but at the same time I wanted to know. I am not ready to give up to this disease! I have just gotten through this and started to recover. I want to know what I need to do to fight it!

I felt like I was struck with a bolt of lightning. I listened to what the genetic counselor had to say about the genetic testing. I started to get teary and then, it was like a bomb was dropped. If the testing came back, positive or negative, I would have to make a decision to either have a left mastectomy, or have an MRI, mammograms, and breast ultrasounds done every six months. If it was positive, I would be in the 40-50 percentiles to have cancer come back in the lung, the bone, or the liver. It was more than I wanted to know. My heart was in my stomach. I cried on the way back to work wondering why all this had to be happening.

I started thinking of the future, knowing that I will always be wondering, "When will it come back, and where?" I thought that maybe, if I would just get angry and scream, that I might feel better. But I couldn't. I just kept saying, "Why now?"

I knew that if I dwelled on this information that I would not be able to live peacefully. It would destroy my marriage and my inner self if I allowed this information to consume me. Dr. Geoffrey was right. I needed to bury my

Debbie Ziemann, RN

head in the sand and just try and forget about it. I could not let it control me. But how was I going to accomplish that? I would have to do some deep searching within myself to find the answer.

I called my husband and told him, and asked him to go with me when the results came back. I didn't think that I would be able to handle it alone. I called Dr. Geoffrey, because if the oncologist felt that a mastectomy was the best treatment, I would need to know what he thought and what he would do. He told me that even though it would be hard, I needed to stick my head in the sand and just not think about this at all. I needed to wait and see what happened first. But if things did go that way, he and his father would take care of me, and he would be there to get me through that also.

He said that he was on vacation until next Thursday, and he went to the office to do some paperwork. He saw a note from Bonnie that I asked him to call me. He said that he was glad that he did. I apologized for calling him when he was on vacation and he said that he was glad that I did. He told me that I wasn't doing anything wrong and that he was always there for me.

Thinking about all this later, I pretty much decided that I would have the tests done every six months, and

SURVIVING BREAST CANCER

if they found anything, it would be caught early and we would deal with it then.

With what I thought was all the major grief behind me, I have set my sights on being a survivor. I have been strong and determined through out this entire ordeal. I have always tried to stay positive. I think that I have done that with a significant amount of grace. I have relied on my faith and spirituality to give me strength. I don't allow anyone to tell me sad stories. I have had enough of sadness. There is nothing we can do about yesterday; it is past. There is nothing that we can do about tomorrow, because it is the future and we do not know what it holds. But we can do something about the present. It is a gift! We need to enjoy every moment, take time for ourselves, and enjoy the gift of life and living.

Chapter Seven
LIFE WILL NEVER BE THE SAME

As I got through the holidays, I realized that I had started to dictate my own state of mind. I was a Survivor! I no longer feared the grief that I felt. I welcomed those moments. I knew that it was all right to have bad days, and I would openly cry. I knew that I needed to reach out to others and share my journey; laughing through the tears. I would not feel guilty. I know that I would never forget the pain and suffering, the loss of my breast, and who I was. I would embrace the memories, the grief, and I would fight to get through it. I would live my life knowing that nothing would ever be the same! As a Survivor, I would openly cry and then say, "I'm okay".

I was disfigured and lopsided. I had no hair. I thought my body was repulsive. How could anyone else not think so, especially my husband? How could it not make a difference? Wayne understood how I felt about having no hair and wearing a wig. He told me that I was beautiful even without a head of hair and reminded me that it would grow back. I was soon able to go without the wig at home.

Because we had not been intimate for several months, and I wanted him to touch me, I had to tell him how I was feeling. I had desire to be with him, but I was not ready for intercourse. One morning, when he was getting ready for work and I was helping him dress (because he had broken his elbow and wrist from a fall at work), I sat beside him on the edge of the bed. I asked him if he were afraid to touch me, because he hadn't done that in so very long. He told me that he wasn't, but he didn't want to hurt me. I told him that it would not hurt, and, in fact, that it was hurting me more that he *didn't*. I needed to be touched, kissed, and held. I told him that I had thought that he found me repulsive. He held me and told me that was not true. He loved me whether I had one or two breasts; he married me because of who I am, on the inside. I was a beautiful person and he loved me more than he ever did before. He thought that he was going to lose me,

SURVIVING BREAST CANCER

and this event had brought us closer together. He said, "It doesn't matter to me. You're *here*, and that is all that matters." I could not live without you, Wayne!

I believe that breast cancer is not good for a relationship, but good relationships can be made stronger by sharing the hardship. I am sure that my husband mourned, had doubts, and missed the old me. My husband was there through all the misgivings. He stood by while I cried and screamed, and he hugged me when I let him get close enough. Our marriage is better and stronger than it ever has been.

When I realized that I was afraid to go to bed with him, I apologized. I told him that I realized what I had been doing, and why. I was afraid that I had hurt him, and I never intended or wanted to do that. I told him that this wasn't just my experience, but it was his also. We had to tell each other what we were thinking and feeling. Even though he said that it didn't matter, he understood why I felt that way. It was hard for me to believe him at first. There was some comfort in his words of love and support. I never felt abandoned. He was always there for me emotionally and spiritually and eventually physically.

Since I didn't like who I was, and what I looked like, I made an effort to see myself differently. I took one part of my body at a time. I would stand in front of the mirror looking at my head without hair and stay there until I found three things that I liked about myself. I would not leave until I found those three things. Once I was able to do that, I looked at myself with my wig on. The harder part came when I had to stand in front of the mirror with breasts that were not symmetrical, one without a nipple. I missed the old breast. It doesn't look like the normal breast. I missed being able to feel the sensation of his hand when he touched my breast. I missed the ability to feel in sensitive areas of my body. I still had a lot of numbness. I would cry but I would not leave that position until I found three things to like.

When I had the implants placed, I was excited, but scared. I wondered if the real breast would look nice and feel normal. I knew that the reconstructed breast would not have any sensation. I took the dressings off to change them and I was amazed at how good they looked. They were nearly the same size. One was a little lower than the other but I was sure that when I was able to wear a bra that no one would be able to tell. I showed my husband and he was happy. He marveled at the work that Dr. Geoffrey had done. As the swelling went down, they looked even better than they had before. I was able to stand in front of the mirror, and not only not cry, but smile. I was happy with the way that I looked. But, I still wanted a nipple and belly button. They are part of our body image, and in order to continue to be comfortable with how I looked to myself, I knew that I needed to have that done.

After Christmas, I had the nipple and belly button constructed. The nipple and breast looked great. Wayne was so excited and told Dr. Geoffrey that he thought that he had done what he thought God could only do. Dr. Geoffrey was happy that we were so pleased.

When I was changing the dressing, I stood in front of the mirror, and I was able to say that I liked what I saw. I easily found three things that I liked about myself and how I looked. Now, an even harder subject had to be approached: I had no libido, and I knew there was nothing that could be done for that. My heart wanted to be intimate, but my body didn't want to respond to my husband's touch. I felt inadequate. I was frustrated because I could not feel the warmth and tenderness of his touch. It frightened me! Would I ever be able to feel that tenderness, that sexual excitement again? I would cry.

Debbie Ziemann, RN

This is normal for women who go through chemotherapy. I had not stopped thinking about sex, but I was afraid. In order to resume our sexual activity, even though talking about sex has always been a problem for me, I knew that I needed to have good communication with my husband. I needed to let him know my fears and sadness about performing, or the inability for my body to respond. I did not want him to think that he was doing something wrong, or not enough. But I needed to feel that closeness that a married couple has during this recovery phase.

A good marriage takes hard work on a daily basis from both partners, under normal circumstances. When a life-threatening event occurs, it is even harder, and there needs to be a lot of understanding. Both partners have to share in the responsibility.

One weekend, Wayne wanted intimacy. I did too! Taking time in foreplay, which we had discussed before, did not happen. He did not touch me, kiss me, or hold me. I was leaving the bedroom to make breakfast, and he said to me to let him know when I was ready. I was hurt and disappointed! I felt inadequate, and the burden of resuming our sex life was now just placed entirely on my

SURVIVING BREAST CANCER

shoulders! How was I ever going to be ready if he wasn't going to help me?

All my fears, in that fleeting moment, came back! I again thought that I looked deformed and mutilated; I was no longer attractive or desirable to him. I got angry because it took so long and it was a struggle to find my confidence and self-esteem, and it was shot down in a matter of seconds! How could he have done this to me? Did he even know what he had done?

I was nervous, and felt very awkward, but I talked to him about going slow and just starting out by making some relaxed time together. We would light candles or burn incense. We spent time kissing and holding one another, and doing entire body touching. We did this one at a time, not at the same time. I needed to be self-centered and tuned into my own feelings, and not be worried about my husband's thoughts or feelings.

My goal was to just enjoy the sensual pleasure. I was not looking to being sexually excited. Not yet, I wasn't ready, because I knew that my body would not respond. I didn't want to become frustrated. We had to do this several times and it relieved the nervousness and pressure of being close.

Even though talking about sex and what I needed for him to do was awkward and embarrassing for me, I knew that good communication was important. This was not the time for embarrassment to silence me. I had to let him know in either words, or by guiding his hand, the touches that I needed. I think that this all came about because being with him was the only thing that made me feel alive. I feel safe and protected in his arms. I remembered feeling like I was melting when he would hold me and I wanted to feel that way again! With the fear of death hanging over my head, I needed that!

We are still working with this process. I still become frustrated at times because my body doesn't respond. My husband is such a gentle "giant." He doesn't say much, but he will try whatever I need to make me comfortable. He has never made me feel self-conscious or embarrassed about how I look, or my inability to respond to his touch. Using this means of helping me to become sexually excited has brought us closer together because we are working to achieve a goal together.

We were very sexually active as any newlywed couple is, and when this event took place, it was like sex was the last thing on either of our minds. But we are now on another plane in our sex life. Holding hands, kissing,

SURVIVING BREAST CANCER

rubbing each other's feet and bodies brings us the closeness that we had before. It will take awhile for my body to respond, but in the meantime, we are enjoying the quiet time together, touching one another. It gives us both pleasure and comfort. We talk and laugh. We can lie in each other's arms and be comforted and content: one of life's "little pleasures."

Chapter Eight

STRUGGLING THROUGH THE GRIEF

*B*eing told that I had breast cancer was like being hit by a Mack Truck! Our breasts are a part of who we are. They determine part of our sexual attractiveness to society, our partners, our spouses, and ourselves. They are a part of our sexual life that gives both our partners pleasure and ourselves. As mothers who nursed their children, we found comfort in knowing that we were giving our baby's natural immunity and good health. They found comfort lying in our arms nestled in our breasts. They found pleasure when they played on our laps and buried their heads between our breasts.

As a nurse, I have seen almost everything. I thought it had made me stronger than a layperson. I was wrong!

Underneath it all, I am still a woman, and the loss was greater than I realized. It was not until I went back to work that I really started having trouble accepting my new body imagine. I had difficulty looking at myself in the mirror. In fact, I couldn't! I had lost my hair from the treatments and I was self-conscious about wearing a wig. I didn't want my husband, or anyone, to see me without hair. I didn't want my husband to see me naked, or even touch me. I was afraid!

The fatigue was, and is, indescribable! No one understands just how dreadful you feel. When the treatments are all over, the effects linger for a year or more. With a trans-flap, or a total mastectomy, the skin is highly sensitive, and there are muscle spasms, and soreness in your arms and chest. This can last a long time. You try to catch up with everything, try to work, and get back to normal, but you can't. There is no "normal"! You cannot meet your own expectations, and if you have gone back to work, you cannot meet your employers. This is when the reality really started to "sink in!" There is lack of total energy, and a kind of weakness throughout your entire body. There is no interest in people and the things that you used to enjoy.

SURVIVING BREAST CANCER

Fatigue comes from worry, the diagnosis, treatment, other medical problems, and all the baggage that you carry – it just hangs on! You don't feel normal, or feel good, but you keep making appointments that your body just cannot meet!

I found that you just have to accept the fatigue. You cannot fight it! It is a sign that your body needs to heal. Your mind and spirit need to heal. I learned to sit and take deep breaths; enjoy the sunset and the moonlight. I had to stop running away from it, and move *into* it, and explore other possibilities. I needed to learn when I felt the most fatigued, and then at those times, try and rest. I had to learn what my stressors were, and learn how to manage those.

Whenever I started to feel overwhelmed with the fatigue or emotions, I would write in my journal. I think that it makes it more real, and by writing, you learn what you need to do to help yourself: just listen to what your body is telling you!

The very act of focusing on my imperfections, as I saw them, was pulling me away from my goal to be a survivor. It stopped me from enjoying and appreciating everything that I have and how things already were.

It is impossible to feel peaceful with your head so full of concerns. For me, the solution to control those fears and concerns was to control the thoughts in my head, before they had a chance to build up momentum. By writing my feelings down in my journal, I could then put them away. There is nothing more important than your own sense of happiness and inner peace and that of your loved ones. Don't waste precious moments of life when there is no way to control the inevitable: whatever that will be!

I had to realize that the peace of mind I wanted and needed had to come from within. I had to learn to live in the present moment! It was where I was at, and where we are – always! I didn't ask for this disease. I realized, in part, that it was there to teach me a lesson, and to teach my husband a lesson, as well.

With soul-searching, I realized where my weaknesses were. I was always so strong and independent, and I never socialized with friends – I kept to myself. Now, I have found that I am not so strong, and that I need my family and friends. I needed to socialize, laughing through my tears, at myself, and to not take life and living so seriously. I needed friends to talk to, to share this journey with, so that I was able to fight through the grief. I found there was more to life than just work, and the hassles of everyday living.

I found that I needed my husband more than I ever did. Some of our arguments in the first few months of our marriage revolved around my independence. Now I am more gentle, and hopefully, more kind. I am very dependent on him. As my life's partner, whom other should I be kinder to than him?

I remember the words that I said to him in our wedding ceremony: "You were a dream, then you became a possibility, and then a reality. You loved me for who I was, for who I am, and, for who I will become. I love you with all my heart, my mind, my body, and my soul." Those few words have more meaning today than they did on one of the happiest days of my life! I had to surrender to the fact that life isn't fair. "Bad things do happen to good people." Surrendering myself to this fact gave me the courage to do my best, one day at a time, resting when I needed to, or going home from work early, because my energy was low and crying if I felt like crying.

Taking one day, and one moment at a time, has taught me to be more flexible instead of so structured. I had expectations of myself, and my body, that I could not meet. I always tried to be happy and confident, and I wouldn't cry because I wanted to appear strong and have people believe I was okay. That thought process doesn't work. It doesn't allow for flexibility in your daily life, and not crying doesn't allow you to heal. It is okay to cry and have a bad day, as many as you need! Any problem can become devastating if you allow it to, but then, you feel out of control when you don't allow yourself some flexibility.

Changing my mood from sadness, feeling despair, and out of control, to one of being happy was difficult. I realized I had to be content and grateful for where I was, at the moment, on this path of renewed health. Life will always be filled with challenges. Declining health as we age is a reality we all face. It is best to admit this to yourself and decide to be happy, in spite of it. There is no way to happiness. Happiness is the way! We have a choice to decide our attitude in response to any given situation. We can look at the bad and be negative, or we can take that situation and learn something from it. I did not need, or even *want*, the cancer and the grief to control me, but for a while it did. With determination and renewed confidence, and emotional and spiritual strength, I am finding my way back home!

I had to gain my sense of personal power. I was able to see myself as a choice maker, and I decided that I would not let cancer make me powerless. It became my source of strength and power. Circumstances, no matter if they are good or bad they may be, reveal who we are. I wanted to reveal that I was a Survivor!

Judy, from our bereavement department, said to me that I was a "wounded warrior." I had been strong and steadfast; I always smiled, and I had a positive attitude. I hadn't really done any grieving until after the surgeries and treatment. I told her it was as if everyone was right there for me when I was getting through the chemotherapy and surgery, but now they were gone. Now is when I started the real grieving process, and I needed my friends the most to talk to, to listen, and to walk this journey with me. It gives strength and hope to be able to share your feelings. Telling people how I felt has helped me find the path to a solution, and to find some comfort, contentment and peace.

When I went back to work and resumed some normal activity, it was assumed that I was all right, and that the worst was over. It's not! The grieving just begins. The hurt is deeper than anyone can imagine or comprehend.

The emotional suffering, on this journey to recovery, has been difficult, to say the least. It has taught me to be humble, grateful, and patient. Accepting breast cancer taught me that life can be more of a dance and less of a battle. I suppose that is part of the philosophy of "go with the flow." I had to learn to make peace with my new body.

To accomplish this sense of wonder, I needed to look for the extraordinary in the ordinary. I had, and have, so much to be grateful for, that I sit in awe. Life is so precious and extraordinary! We need to take time to "smell the roses" along the way. It gives all new meaning to "living life to the fullest" and "enjoying one day at a time", one experience after another.

I was getting a massage one evening and read an read an article about Laughter Therapy. There was a quote by a from James Green, a longtime AIDS survivor; "if you go around in an angry state of consciousness you are not "healing." While I was getting the massage, I lay there, with my eyes closed, and began to think deeply about what it was that he said and what the article revealed.

I realized that laughing at adversity helps by empowering you and it broadens your perspective. I wanted to read more about laughter therapy. I went to the bookstore and there were an immense number of books on laughter therapy. What I found was that laughing not only creates several chemical reactions, but also that my mind cannot hold two separate opposing thoughts at the same time. When we are happy and laughing, the body is producing a chain of immune-enhancing chemicals, and the healing is much more profound.

If you have ever been to Arizona, the freeway is a parking lot at specific times of the day; going to work and on the way home. I absolutely hated the drive home, especially. To drive twenty-two miles, at five o'clock, can take anywhere from one and a half to two hours! So I gave this laughter theory a try: I just started laughing out loud. I thought of things that normally would make me upset, and I looked for the ridiculous in them, and just heartily laughed! To my surprise, I felt better. I wasn't as tired when I got home. I was in a better mood and my muscles did not hurt so much.

I tried this when I was just having an emotionally low day. I went outside and thought about why I was down, and then I started to laugh about it because I could not change what had happened to me. Although I was crying, I was still laughing. I did this for twenty minutes without realizing it. To my surprise, I felt better once again. Every day, at least twice a day, I spend fifteen minutes laughing. It may not be about anything at all; I might have simply thought of something funny, or, I just laughed at myself for being so enclosed into my negative thoughts about this journey that I am taking.

Chapter Nine
A SPECIAL CHRISTMAS, 2004

It was the week of Christmas, and although I was feeling much better since I had been off the Tamoxifen, I was anxious about my sons (and their girlfriends) coming. I did not know how they were going to react when they saw me. I had decorated the house to make the fantasy world that they had known since childhood. Wayne had more food than you can imagine! He always wants to be sure that they have plenty of food. He makes me laugh because he says that they are growing boys!

I was still wearing the wig. I looked tired, and I was. I had been crying all the time and I didn't want to cry when they were here. I had always been their pillar of strength: they never saw me cry, and when I was sick, I always continued to do what needed to be done. Now, I had no control over my feelings and I couldn't do much without being fatigued.

Evan and his girlfriend, whom we had not met yet, would be here first. Now, I had to face a stranger with all my imperfections. Evan had always been inquisitive about how I was feeling, how Wayne was doing, and strangely enough, he would ask personal questions about our intimate life. One day, he just point blank asked if we were having sex! Hurriedly he said, "I know that is a strange question for a son to ask, but it's an important part of a relationship." I was honest, in some sense, telling him that the surgeries and the chemotherapy had taken away the desire. But, that we have, once in awhile, been intimate without having intercourse.

Evan and Carli drove from California and it was a great greeting. Evan ran to me calling me "Mommie" and held on to me tightly. He introduced me to Carli and I gave her a hug. She is a very beautiful young girl; two years younger than Evan, but what a wonderful mind. She is full of passion and compassion, and intelligent. How lucky I feel that Evan has found such a wonderful partner to share life with.

Surviving Breast Cancer

Evan picked up Aaron at the airport, and when I got home from work, he came out to meet me. He smiled and said, "Hi, Mama," and he held me tightly. Tears started to well in my eyes. He did not mention my wig and didn't say anything about my breasts when he hugged me. I didn't know if they felt normal to anyone when we hugged. Not even Wayne had ever said. He took the things that I brought home with me and we went inside. I hugged everyone because I had to leave for work before anyone was up.

I was off the day Brady and his girlfriend flew in. I was very nervous about seeing him. He was still angry about the cancer. We picked them up. They had had a very bad flight. Neither he nor Lindsey enjoyed flying. Lindsey, in fact, is petrified! Brady was upset because he didn't know how to help Lindsey, so the initial reunion was not what I had expected.

When we were all at home, things settled in. The boys hugged me. Brady came up to me and hugged me, holding on tightly. He said that he was sorry for not coming when I probably needed him, but that he just couldn't. I told him that it was okay.

129

We were all in the living room, and Aaron asked if my hair was growing. I told them that it was and moved the wig back a little so that they could see. They told me to take it off; that I didn't need to wear it. I felt my stomach sink. I mustered up the courage and took it off. To my amazement, all of them said that it looked good. I was thinking, "Yeah, right! You're just saying that, so I don't feel bad." Later, however, they would rub their hands through what hair I did have, and I knew then it was okay.

What happened next, I am sure would make most mothers angry, but for me, it was a way for me to know that they had accepted what had happened to me. All the kids and I were in the kitchen, and Brady came up to me and touched my breast, and asked, "How are the boobies?" I asked them all if they wanted to see what the end result was. To my surprise they did! So, I lifted up my top and showed them. Their eyes filled with amazement! Aaron, who had seen the breast at its worst, just could not believe how great it looked. I explained the whole procedure that was done. Aaron then wanted to see my belly because he had helped me with the dressings. He told everyone that both of them looked great, a big improvement from what he had seen before.

They needed to see for themselves that I was all right! I needed them to see so that I would be okay. So I would not be afraid, or embarrassed, around them. This gave me the opportunity to tell them, all together, about my anxiety and my fear about them being here for the first time since all this had happened. They smiled and hugged me, and told me that I was their Mom, and that they loved me for who I am, not what I look like. The anxiety was gone, and we were all able to relax and enjoy each other.

At Christmas Eve dinner, Wayne made the comment that I had been through a lot this year. I told him that he had, too: that we *all* had a difficult year and been through a lot. Every one of us had to struggle through this, in our own way. Brady raised his wine glass for a toast. "We are glad that you are here, and we love you. We love you both!"

Christmas 2004 will always be a "Special Christmas." I was alive and free of cancer, and spending the holiday with my family. My heart was lifted when I knew that I didn't need to be afraid that they would be disgusted with how I looked. I think that even Wayne was relieved when he saw how they felt, and what they had said, because we even seemed closer than a week or two before. I believe

Debbie Ziemann, RN

that it was the spirit of the holiday, of God's Angels, who freed my soul and heart from the anxiety and despair that I had been feeling. I was not afraid to live life anymore. I knew that I would be okay! I would be a Survivor!

To Hope Is To Fly.

To Fly is to Dream
To Dream is to Believe
To Believe is to Do.
To Do is to give Hope
To give Hope Is to fight the fight of Angels

Chapter Ten
REDISCOVERING MYSELF

Today, I'll look within and seek to please myself.

*I*n the fall of each year, caterpillars work hard to make their cocoons for the winter. As spring begins to arrive, they struggle to form a new life. The result is a beautiful butterfly, fighting to reach the warmth of the sun, and to take flight into the new world. So it is, with the breast cancer survivor.

We struggle and fight to get through that first year of tests, surgeries, chemotherapy, loss of hair, fatigue, and acceptance of our new body image, and hot flashes and night sweats; the emotional roller coaster that we have been on. As it comes to a close, we find that we are still struggling and wondering, "When will it all end?"

Debbie Ziemann, RN

I am not sure that it ever will.

> Eyes, what are they? Colored glass,
> Where reflections come and pass.
> Open windows – by them sit
> Beauty, Learning, Love and Wit.
> *- Mary Elizabeth Coleridge*

The fight to survive is difficult to say the least! We have to work at accepting our new body and how it looks to us. How we appear in other's eyes can become an obsession. Do they see me as I see myself? Or do they see the real me? Is that worse, or is it better? I wonder if their eyes are a mirror, in which I will find my own reflection. Or, are they the windows through which I can touch the spirit of those I love? If we esteem ourselves, we won't worry about other's opinions. Of course, we want to be respected and loved by those we love. We want to be accepted as a fellow traveler on life's journey, this difficult journey that we must travel as a breast cancer survivor. But our main concern is our own spiritual growth – and it will be the key to how we are perceived. We miss our breast (or breasts) that we lost. We miss the ability to feel the touch of our spouse or partner. We have to relearn how to enjoy and let go of our fear of having sex again. When we look in the mirror, we see a new growth of hair that is different in color and texture, and we wish that it would grow faster. The fatigue that we have doesn't allow us to enjoy life and living.

We see a reflection of someone that we are not familiar with, and wonder where that person is, who has been so transformed. We are reminded every day of what has happened, and we wish that it would just go away. Our emotions can lead us to the depths of despair that only we can understand, and then we can be on "top of the world" in the same day. No one understands this emotional roller coaster that we must endure.

There have been days that I did not know who I was, or where this new life had taken me, and I continued to struggle with my self-confidence and my self-esteem. My priorities seemed to change on a daily basis. I was confused and lost. I was overwhelmed with work, and with life in general. There were times when I felt like running away, because the burden of finding my new identity rested solely on my shoulders.

I am just starting to do the things that renewed my spirit before I was diagnosed with breast cancer. Even those things are still a struggle to do. I continue to have a sense of urgency that I do not understand. With soul-searching, I am sure that I will find a meaning to that

Debbie Ziemann, RN

urgency. Taking one moment at a time is the best thing that I can do. I do not worry about those things that I cannot change.

When we return to work, our co-workers think that everything is back to normal. What they do not understand is that there is no "normal" anymore! Nothing will ever be the same! The struggle will always be with us; there is no letting go. Your co-workers will not allow you to share your journey anymore; when *this* is the time that you need to talk the most. They expect you to be happy, every day: full of energy and life. We are trying to find our "new identity" and they are not there to help us.

Our supervisors place expectations on us that our minds and bodies are not able to meet. We have learned to listen to our bodies, and not set expectations that we cannot meet. With our priorities changing, we do not know where our life is taking us. We find ourselves being anxious and frightened. The instinct of "fight or flight" comes to the surface, and we end up in another turmoil because we do not know what to do, where to go, what to say, or what not to say.

Our loved ones have a desire to move back to, or find, that normalcy that we had before. They do not know, or understand how, to help us. They are men and they are the "fix it" people. They become frustrated, worried, and scared. They just don't know how to give us the comfort and support that we need. They are frightened that they are going to lose us: emotionally and physically. Men do not talk about their fears. They are to be strong and they do not cry.

They are the protectors; the ones who must maintain the household, and they take care of the finances. That is stressful for both partners. If there is a financial strain in the home that may be where his focus is: his focus may not be on understanding and supporting your loss of self.

With our fears that they see us as deformed, we may push them away, just when they need intimacy. We may not even realize that we are doing it. It becomes a vicious cycle that we create, and then, we don't understand our partner. Our confidence and self-esteem plummet and we withdraw.

I was feeling out of place; not knowing where I was going. I didn't want to work. I dreaded going to work, every day. Fatigue made it nearly impossible for me to do my job adequately. (Or, at least that is how I felt.) I was afraid to see patients, and just the thought of driving to a home to complete a supervisory visit made me anxious. I began to think that I needed to make a career change.

I went on a business trip for the management team in February. I remember feeling overwhelmed as I ran some errands and packed to leave. I started to cry as I drove to pick my husband up at work, so that he could take me to the airport. I realized that I was afraid to go without him. He is my strength, and he gave me courage on a daily basis. My husband was the only one who understood my fatigue. Holding his hand as we walked in public places gave me the confidence that I needed to hold my head up, to look people in the eyes, and to smile.

As we drove to the airport, I started to cry. I told him that I didn't want to go and why. He took my hand and told me that I would be all right. If it was too much for me I should get on a plane and come home. He would be here for me. He held me tightly at the airport, and he reassured me that I was all right.

I was exhausted when we arrived. The rest of the group was waiting in the hotel for us. Everyone else wanted to go out and walk around, and then get something to eat. I felt that I had to go along; that I needed to participate.

Walking down Bourbon Street, I became so exhausted that I could barely stand up. Every muscle in my body seemed to ache.

We went to dinner, and then two of us walked back to the hotel, while the others did some sight-seeing. I found myself looking down at the street as I walked, so that I would not make eye contact with anyone. When we arrived at the hotel, I went directly to my room, took a shower, and went to sleep.

I didn't sleep well. I was tossing and turning most of the night. I was worried with facing strangers from other hospices and the corporate managers. I didn't take my wig with me because that is not who I am now, but neither was the short, curly hair! I kept telling myself that I should have brought the wig, but I am always wondering if people knew that it wasn't my real hair. I realized that I was making myself into a victim, and not a Survivor. Because of the fatigue, I was afraid that my co-workers would not understand why I was not able to go out every evening. I didn't want them to think that I didn't want to be with them, or be a part of them.

We finished early the first day of the meeting, and we were to meet in the lobby to walk to dinner with everyone.

I went up to my room to rest, so that I would be able to stay up with everyone, and I could participate in the sightseeing after dinner. I fell asleep, and woke up after everyone had left for dinner. I was hurt because they left without seeing if I was going, or even if I was all right. I even thought that they may be embarrassed about my appearance. Tears ran down my face. I didn't feel a part of hospice anymore. I could not see myself working with them, and I thought that I needed to resign.

I met with one of the speakers, regarding the personality test that we had to take prior to going to the meeting. I asked if being diagnosed with breast cancer, and trying to re-identify who I now was, would influence the results. I told her that I even considered making a career change. She looked at the results, and said that I am right where I should be. That maybe, there were certain personalities at work who were making me feel that I needed to change. She reminded me that re-learning who I am takes awhile, after going through a life-threatening event, and that I needed to be patient with myself.

She asked who I saw when I looked in the mirror. I told her that I wondered who that person was and where the old person had gone. She reaffirmed that I am a new person. She said that the disease and the threat of my mortality had changed how I look at different aspects of life, but that the old me was still there. She also asked if things that used to drive me crazy still did. I told her that they didn't. She then told me that, because of this unfortunate event in my life, I have taken on a new outlook. She explained that even though my priorities have changed, the old me was still there. I was learning to love the old self, while accepting the new identity.

That evening, I thought about what she had said to me. I realized that to recover emotionally would take longer than I expected. I learned to accept that the people with whom I worked and I were all going through the grieving process, but at different times and rates. I should not expect to be through the grieving process in less than a year.

I came back from the meeting feeling somewhat better about who I now was, realizing that who I was prior to cancer was still who I am now. But, I had come back with new worries; I found a small lump on my left breast; the right breast was aching; and the implant seemed to have moved from its normal position. The belly button was healing, but I found another area inside that was not there before. I called Dr. Geoffrey's office and made an appointment for the next day.

I told Dr. Geoffrey what was happening and apologized for panicking. He told me that I should have called him when I got back on Sunday. He examined the right breast and said that the tissue was softer than before. He was concerned that I may have broke the pocket, and that the implant may have moved, but it was still all right. He looked at the belly button and told me that I should no longer pack it, and that I should just leave it closed. If it looked okay, then he would not do anything with it, unless I wanted him to.

At this point, I don't want anything else done. I already had one surgery scheduled for March, and I did not want to think about another. I showed him the lump on the left breast. I told him that I just had to know what he thought. He told me that he understood, and yes, I did need to know. I started to cry. He examined the mass and said that he was sure that it was either dead fat tissue or scar tissue. He promised that he would follow it closely, and if it grew he would remove it. I told him that I was going to have a mammogram and a breast ultrasound the following day, and he asked to have those results faxed to him.

I was nervous about having the mammogram and ultrasound done. It was a year ago that I had the first mammogram. After they were through with the tests, I asked if everything was all right, knowing that they would not tell me the results. They said that the doctor would have to tell me the results. The technician left the room, and I broke into tears. The anxiety of waiting for the results was overwhelming. I cried on the way home and decided that I would call Dr. Geoffrey's office, to ask the nurse if she would ask him to call me with the results when they received them. She told me that she would have him call me. I felt some relief because I knew that he would call me before the week was over. Fear of the unknown is haunting! I took some deep breaths and started to relax. I was going to be positive and not negative. I was going to let the universe take care of itself!

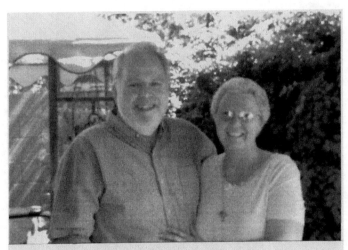

Above: Wayne & Debbie Ziemann today
Below: Wayne & Debbie with Yoda & Missey

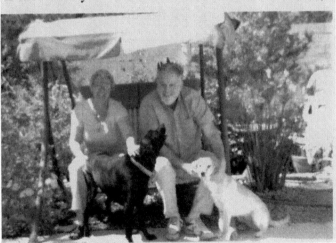

Chapter Eleven
I'm Okay!

My efforts on my own behalf are never wasted.

We are reminded, every day, of what has happened to us, and we wish that it would just go away. Our emotions can lead us to the depths of sorrow that only we can understand, and then we can be on the "top of the world" in the same day.

There is one person, and only one, on whose life we can have a strong, positive influence, and that is ourselves. What is more: we *deserve* our own support. We richly repay our efforts on our own behalf. Anything we can do for ourselves will stay with us; the more we learn, the wiser we will become.

We really have not lost the person we were; we are still here. We grieve for the loss of someone who we have been comfortable with, for however many years we have lived. We have lost that person's humor, that person's appearance, and that person's body…but we are still there. We have had to endure the pain of several months of surgery, treatment, and the struggle to accept a new body, all while fighting through the emotions to survive. But that person, that we thought that we lost, is still there!

We really are no different than we were. We just need to find that person again. We can love, we can laugh, we can cry, and we can feel compassion, anger, and relief. It is all right to feel you have lost the person that you were. It is part of the grieving process.

It has been eleven months since I was diagnosed with breast cancer. I will continue to fight this battle to find my new identity, but I know that the old person is still there. The person is in my heart, my mind, and my soul: that does not change! What have changed are my priorities; how I look at living life, and what I want to give to life. We cannot expect life to give us anything! It is all about compassion and love: loving others and ourselves, and sharing our journey with those who do not understand.

SURVIVING BREAST CANCER

It is through our bodies that we experience life. Our senses allow us to rediscover the pleasure and rewards of being in our bodies, of being in the present, and of appreciating our surroundings. I found that if I used all of my senses - sight, sound, smell, taste, and touch - that it was a doorway, inviting me to rediscover the pleasure and reward of being within my new body. If I stayed within myself, I was not present to those lives around me.

I worried about the future, and ignored how to heal myself. I did not allow myself to feel complete. I realized that I had to reconnect with life; where my heart opened and my feelings flow. That was the territory of the present and a realm of the heart where I wasn't going because I was too tired, too afraid, and this journey was too arduous. This journey I am on is demanding, but it can also be fulfilling.

When I become emotionally charged, I have learned to step back and not react. I breathe deeply and engage all of my senses. I awaken the body and mind, bringing them together as one, so that I am not running away, but *charging* into life's experience. I was learning to find the abundance of love within myself, and others. If I listened with my whole body, I was able to gain a perspective that I would not otherwise have been able to do.

I found that by doing this, I was able to cling to the pleasant experiences and avoid the unpleasant ones, and to realize that both are a part of life. When I committed myself to living through all of my senses, I became committed to living through my heart. I committed myself to self-love, and love of others. Doing so then became an expression of who I am, and my actions then took on integrity. I became less confused, less stuck in a place of being lost. I became more curious, more adventurous, more playful, and more eager to feel and try new things. Our senses and bodies are a part of one another. To be able to experience those, I found the beauty within myself, and the power to free myself to be who I am.

Sonia Osorio, in *Body Sense*, gives some awakening suggestions:

"Communicate your desires directly and honestly, listen compassionately – the person speaking is a part of you, have the courage to be fearful, have the strength to be vulnerable, have the wisdom to be foolish, have the maturity to play, and redefine the roles of sensuality and pleasure as something other than sex."

I will be Okay; I am Okay! I have bad days, and I still cry. That is all right. Life will never be the same. The first year, I think, will be the hardest, following the diagnosis and treatment. There will always be the worry that it may come back. It will be a thought that I will have every day. Every time I am not feeling well, or if I find a lump, I will wonder if it is back. I will always be reminded, every day, what happened when I undress or look at my hair.

The fatigue will probably last as long as it takes get through the whole ordeal, which took me nearly a year, because of all the complications and surgeries that I had to have. I have started massage therapy, and very mild exercise, and I am trying to listen to my body when it says its time to rest. Wayne doesn't understand the fatigue, but he is learning to be patient with me. I am learning that I can't do all the things that I want or need to do. Working takes all my energy, and I have little left over for what needs to be done at home.

Eating better, and taking care of myself are both important parts of healing and trying to prevent reoccurrence: I avoid foods with preservatives; I eat more vegetables and fruit; I eat less red meat; I drink plenty of water (up to a gallon a day); I don't drink much caffeine anymore.

I have been able to accept my new body, although I know that my husband is still having problems. We are working on that together. He is still afraid to touch the reconstructed breast: afraid that he will hurt me. I am confident that our sexual life will improve as long as we keep the lines of communication open. We need to let each other know what it is that we need the other to do to satisfy each other. We need both patience and time. We need to make the time to be together, because there is never a right, or good, time to share intimacy.

My hair is growing back, but I still wear my wig. I think it is because of pride and vanity that I continue to wear it. My husband, sons, and friends at work feel that I should stop wearing it. They tell me that my hair looks good and is cute. "Cute", at fifty-two years young, does not sound appropriate. I just am not ready to go without the wig yet! That is okay but I think that it will happen soon.

We have a male nurse who lost his sister to breast cancer. One day we were outside, and he came up to me, when I was wearing a cap, and told me that I should just take it off. He told me about his sister and how he told her that he wanted to see her head. He told her that she had a beautiful shaped head, and that she was still as beautiful as before she lost her hair. Then, he took my hand and said that I was an attractive woman. He noticed that I always carried myself proudly, and he understood. He thought that I, too, should take off the cap, and stop wearing the wig, and I would see more smiles than I ever thought possible. I know that one of these days I will be confident enough in my new identity to stop wearing it, but that day has not come yet. I am getting there. Little did I know that within a few days of that conversation, I would not be placing that mop on my head. And yes, he was right: there were lots of smiles!

Wayne and I went to dinner and I decided that I would try not wearing the wig. I walked into the restaurant, holding my spouse's hand tightly. I followed him to the table, looking down at the floor. I thought that everyone was looking at me and staring. I couldn't enjoy the meal. But, I wasn't ready to give up yet. We went out for lunch the next day, and I was able to walk with my head up, and look at people. I was still uncomfortable, but I didn't withdraw. I knew then that it was time to go to work without the wig.

I dressed, and stood standing in front of the mirror. Tears came to my eyes because I was afraid to go to work without the wig: some people only knew me with that mop. I was afraid that people would laugh and stare, and talk about me behind my back. I thought that they would

Debbie Ziemann, RN

laugh at me and think that I looked awful, or ridiculous. But I stood tall and erect, took a deep breath and told myself that I was going to do this. That this is who I am, at this moment! Everyone said they liked my hair. They smiled and ran their fingers through it. It made me uncomfortable the first day. As the days passed, it became easier.

I have found that my priorities have changed. I no longer worry about cleaning the house. I am lucky that we can have someone do that for me. I am taking time to relearn how to enjoy the things that I used to do. I used to get up every morning and play the radio or my favorite CDs. I haven't done that for nearly a year. Now, I am starting to do that all over. I play CDs in my car, and play those that made me feel good. When I start feeling down, I listen to some relaxation CDs, or I read some short books that make me laugh.

I continue to write in my journal, because I still have bad days. It is so helpful to put it into words and find the answer to my sadness. I find a path to peace and contentment. I am no longer afraid to have a bad day and to cry. I have learned to laugh through my tears. I am sure that I will continue to cry when I talk to someone about this journey, but I realize that the journey has been a good one. I have learned who my true friends are. There are true friends, and then there are "friends" who are really just acquaintances. I will treasure my true friends because they were there for me when I needed to talk, to cry, and to be hugged.

I have gone from a person who didn't like to be hugged to one that gives hugs to people every day! I am not afraid to tell people that I love them. I used to think that telling someone you loved them was reserved only for your family and partner. It is not! It is the extraordinary in the ordinary that allows you to feel free to share your feelings and your life. We cannot be afraid to share what is in our hearts or the compassion that we have for others. Love is the bridge that leads us to happiness.

I have been allowed to share my life with those who are close to me and those that were not. I made some new friends this past year. I found support from co-workers I didn't know very well. I am also sharing my life with those who have taken the opportunity to read this book.

Working in hospice is a wonderful career in nursing. The people I work with have shown the uniqueness of the hospice philosophy — accepting others where they are in

Debbie Ziemann, RN

life, not passing judgment on their past, and helping them go through the end-of-life process.

I am not dying, but they had compassion for their co-worker, whether it was someone that I worked closely with on a daily basis, or someone that I hardly knew, or didn't know at all; they were there for me to talk to, allowing me to cry, allowing me to share my journey so that I could heal emotionally and spiritually.

It is unfortunate that I will have to give up my career in hospice at some point. Going through this experience has made me a better hospice nurse. I can understand our patients', and their family's, emotional pain and grief. I understand how to help them move forward in their grieving process. However, it limits my ability to heal myself. I know that someday I will be able to return to being a hospice nurse.

I still have another loss to deal with. That is the loss of the patient-doctor relationship that I have with Dr. Geoffrey Leber. He has been a vital part of my support system. It will be a good loss, but a loss, nonetheless. I will grieve and cry. Today, I am not ready for that loss. I have shared this with him as I have shared many times how much I have appreciated his comfort and support.

People do come and go in our lives, at special times, with a special purpose. Often, for a purpose, that we don't understand. I consider myself very lucky to know why this special man was chosen to be my plastic surgeon.

My husband does not understand the emotional bond that I have with Dr. Geoffrey. I think that he is jealous at times. He was sitting at the computer one night and said that he didn't know how he felt about him. He couldn't explain why. I held Wayne and told him that I loved him, and that he is the most important part of me. He stood by me and held my hand. We are getting through this together. He had given me the strength and determination to fight this and survive. No one else would accept the deformities I have now. They would not see me the way he does: the person that I am on the inside, loving me for who I am.

I have grown spiritually and found a connection between my body, my mind and my soul. There are no answers to the age-old question of suffering. I cling to the spiritual principle in life...

Debbie Ziemann, RN

Suffering...

Gives meaning to the meaningless
Hope to our hopelessness
Reason to our senselessness
Purpose to our aimlessness
Strength to our Weakness
Courage to our Faintheartedness
Blessed deliverance from our Bitterness
- Author Unknown

Hope, reason, purpose, strength and courage help balance the pain, which can remove the sharp sting from our suffering and waste our sorrows. I see myself as a grain of wheat that has been crushed and buried, and in a sense, it dies...only to rise again into new life. For survivors of breast cancer, our old life is gone and we now have a new life. We learn to live day-by-day, moment-by-moment. We enjoy the extraordinary in the ordinary. We laugh through our tears. We know that nothing will ever be normal again.

SURVIVING BREAST CANCER

I'm Free

Don't grieve for me, for now I'm free
I'm following the path god laid for me.
I took His hand when I heard him call
I turned my back and left it all.

I could not stay another day
To laugh, to love, to work, or play.
Tasks left undone must stay that way.
I found that place at the close of day.

If my parting has left a void
Then fill it with remembered joy.
A friendship shared, a laugh, a kiss.
Ah yes, these things, I too, will miss.

Be not burdened with times of sorrow.
I wish you the sunshine of tomorrow.
My life's been full, I savored much.
Good friends good time, a loved ones touch.

Perhaps my time seemed all too brief;
Don't lengthen it now with undue grief.
Life up your heart and share with me
God wanted me now; He set me Free.

- Author unknown

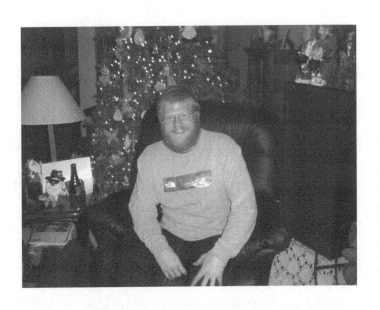
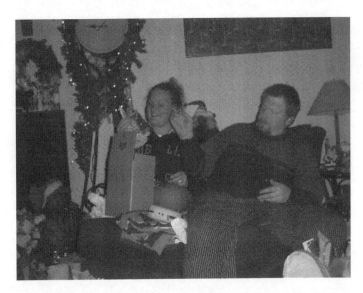

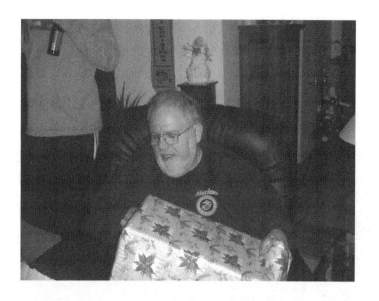
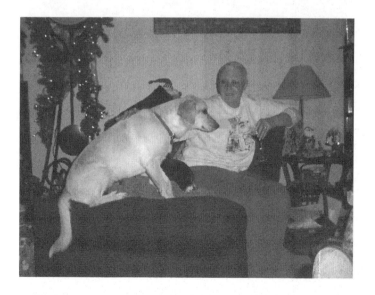

ABOUT THE AUTHOR

Originally from Ohio, Debbie raised her three sons and moved to Arizona in 1997. After completing nursing school in Toledo, Ohio, in 1973, she worked in critical care for eighteen years. She then became a director of nursing in long-term care for another twelve years. More recently, she became part of a hospice organization that provides comfort and support through the end-of-life process for those who wish die at home in the presence of their families. Shortly after she remarried in 2002, she was diagnosed with breast cancer. This is her story of survival. It is the story of her will, her spirit, and her determination to turn this frightening experience into a gift; the ability to celebrate a new life, and a new awareness of herself and the beauty around her. She shares this experience with those who are starting this journey, to help them realize that life is just beginning!

Made in the USA
Lexington, KY
11 March 2017